D1230557

A SICK LIFE

A SICK LIFE

TLC 'n Me: Stories from On and Off the Stage

Tionne "T-BOZ" Watkins

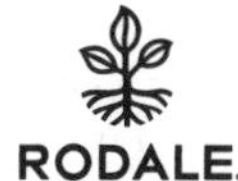

RODALE.

RODALE
wellness

Live happy. Be healthy. Get inspired.

Sign up today to get exclusive access to our authors, exclusive bonuses, and the most authoritative, useful, and cutting-edge information on health, wellness, fitness, and living your life to the fullest.

Visit us online at RodaleWellness.com
Join us at RodaleWellness.com/Join

Rodale books may be purchased for business or promotional use or for special sales. For information, email: BookMarketing@Rodale.com.

Printed in the United States of America
Rodale Inc. makes every effort to use acid-free ♾, recycled paper ♻.

Photographs courtesy of the author

Library of Congress Cataloging-in-Publication Data
is on file with the publisher.

ISBN 978-1-62336-860-9 hardcover
ISBN 978-1-63565-262-8 international paperback
ISBN 978-1-63565-212-3 signed hardcover

Distributed to the trade by Macmillan

2 4 6 8 10 9 7 5 3 1 hardcover
2 4 6 8 10 9 7 5 3 1 international paperback

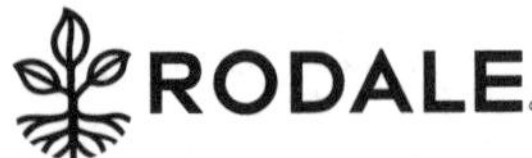

Follow us @RodaleBooks on

We inspire health, healing, happiness, and love in the world.
Starting with you.

I hope my words can be a reign of hope
to anyone who needs them.
And to Ressie, Donnie, Grandma,
and every fallen angel from any disease!

CONTENTS

INTRODUCTION

I believe everything in life happens for a reason. You are meant to be wherever you end up and whoever you become. I was meant to be Tionne "T-Boz" Watkins, a singer, dancer, philanthropist, creator, writer, daughter, mother, sister, and friend. I've spent much of my life in TLC, the world's biggest-selling American girl group of all time. I hear our songs, like "Waterfalls" and "Creep," playing all the time. They're songs that people refer to as timeless and iconic, which is an amazing feeling. Together with Rozonda "Chilli" Thomas and Lisa "Left Eye" Lopes, I created a legacy with TLC. We broke new ground and took down old barriers. We sold millions of albums and inspired millions of fans.

TLC has been an essential aspect of my life, but it's only one part of it. Behind the scenes I've experienced so much. I've dealt with a lifelong illness, sickle cell disease, and I've had dozens of health scares over the years. I gave birth to my daughter, Chase, against medical odds, and recently adopted my son named Chance. Both of them came into my life at very different times and they both felt like miracles—which you'll hear all about later. I'm raising them as a single mother, just like my own mom. I've suffered tragedies and encountered the death of loved ones. I've become a strong, independent woman who refuses to back down.

Over the years, I've learned that there's an upside to everything. You might think your story is the worst and that no one can relate, but there's always someone who's going through the same thing as you—if not worse. My story belongs to me, but I hope it can help those who read it. I hope that my ups and downs and my struggles will make you feel like you're not alone. If I can survive, I know others can, too.

I feel like all my hardships and all my pain have happened for a reason, whatever that reason is. Living with a scary disease has made me a fighter. It's taught me to push forward and look for the positive things in life. Maybe I've gone through all of this and learned these lessons so I could share them and make a difference. Maybe, as you read this, my story can help you.

CHAPTER 1

Two Stories, One Life

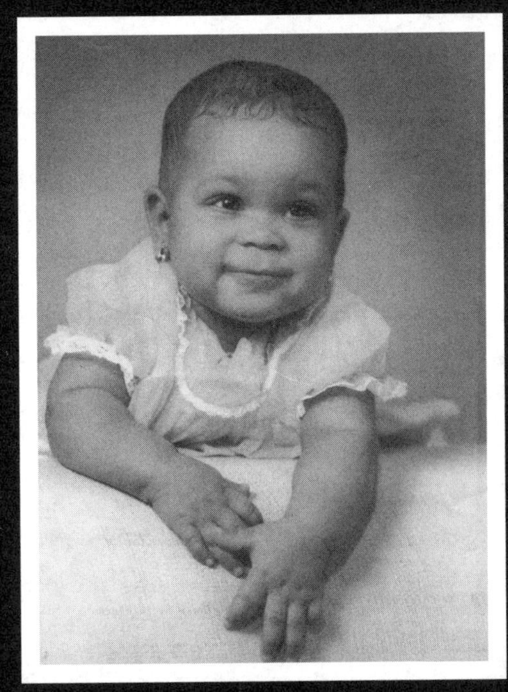

When you perform, there's something that happens right before you go onstage. It's almost magical, like becoming an entirely other person. Before you step out in front of the crowd, you transform into someone else. So, for much of my life, I've been two people. I have been myself, Tionne Watkins, a girl from Atlanta by way of Des Moines, with big dreams and a lifelong illness I've refused to let define me.

But I've also been T-Boz, one third of TLC, the world's biggest girl group. I've had dual stories, but they've both been part of the same life. I have a routine I do when I transform into T-Boz. It's always the same. I look down, rock, pace the floor, and then get really quiet and tune everything out. When I look up, I'm T-Boz. It's an important centering process because music and dance are where I best express myself. It's where my ideas about the world and society and myself can be brought together to create something bigger. For me, music is everything—it makes you feel good, through the positive experiences and the negative ones, and TLC's tracks have always been songs everyone can relate to in some way.

When TLC formed in 1990, we had no idea our music would become so massive. Our second album, *CrazySexy-Cool*, is one of only a few diamond-certified albums ever in the US, selling over 10 million copies, and it was included on *Rolling Stone*'s list of the 500 Greatest Albums of All Time. We won five Grammys, out of 17 total nominations, and we earned four No. 1 singles and ten Top 10 singles. We saw the sort of musical, commercial, and critical success that is rare for artists now, and I still marvel at how that was possible.

During those decades, as TLC formed and grew and exploded into the world, I stayed T-Boz as much as possible when I was in the public eye. I never fully drew back the curtain or revealed what happened behind the scenes, especially on TV or in magazine interviews. I didn't want the press to know everything or to uncover too much of my personal life. I've always been genuine and open with our fans, of course, but I needed to keep some things to myself.

If you see who I am on both sides of the coin, both as Tionne and as T-Boz, you'll understand who I am and how I became a strong, independent woman who refuses to believe anything is impossible. Although T-Boz is an important part of me, I'm clear that I was born Tionne and I'll die Tionne. T-Boz is someone I created, like an alter ego, and I know how to leave her onstage when I go home—unlike some celebs.

On April 26, 1970, I was born Tionne Tenese Watkins to James and Gayle Watkins in Des Moines, Iowa. I came into the world with sickle cell disease, a genetic blood disorder, although my parents didn't know exactly what it was until later. I was sick from the moment I arrived, crying from pain and unable to voice what was ailing me. My dad left me and my mama when I was 3. He was a singer and a trumpet player, and wanted to pursue his musical career in Florida, so my parents separated. I always wanted my father's love and attention, and for those first 3 years we were really close. He took me to Smitty's Donuts and his nickname for me was "Little Vietnam" because I used to run around like I was crazy. Once I got into his band's beer, drank some of it out of the can, ran around in circles, and then passed out. I always thought my dad was in Earth, Wind & Fire because his band would play in our basement and sing "Keep Your Head to the Sky."

My mama raised me on her own, working as many jobs as necessary to give me the best life possible. She always told me I could be whatever I wanted to be, and she always stood by me when I was in pain. Both of my parents could sing, so I think music was in my blood from the beginning. Before they separated, they made an album together, but the record label ran off with the money. My mama's song was "I Don't Care No More" and my daddy's was "Baby Think It Over." Boy, could they sing. And, as it turned out, I could, too.

What I wanted to be, as you'll come to see, was a performer. I was meant for the stage. Singing and dancing came naturally to me, and I loved the feeling of giving something back to an audience. Music can make you feel safe and connected, and it can give you a reason to keep going through any struggle or hardship. Every time I sing and dance, I know I am helping someone. I help them feel less alone. I know this because I have felt alone. I have been consumed with the sense that I'm struggling solo, that no one else seems to understand the pain or challenges I've faced. But the truth is that we all go through bad times, just as we all go through good ones. None of us are alone in that. While my fans may not share my exact struggles and some may not deal with a serious illness like sickle cell disease, I believe there's something everyone can take away from my story. There are different levels of pain, but pain is pain, even though we all handle it differently. It can hurt no matter where it comes from. But if you have a positive attitude and you embrace your own strength, it can help you get past that pain or learn how to cope with it.

My life story is very much linked to sickle cell disease, an incurable blood disorder. The disease, sometimes known as SCD, is hereditary, passed from parents to children in their genes. If a child is born with sickle cell, it means that they've inherited two abnormal hemoglobin genes, one from each parent. It's not something you can catch or develop later in life; it's with you from the moment you come into existence. Sickle cell disease changes the shape of your red blood cells. Instead of being round, like normal red blood cells, SCD cells are curved into a crescent shape (hence the term *sickle*) and can't hold on to oxygen the right way. Because of this, the cells can't get where they need to go, so you can have a stroke, suffer organ failure, or die. It's the sort of thing some people have heard about, but no one ever really seems to know quite what it is.

Although you may not be that familiar with it, sickle cell disease is not uncommon. In fact, it is the most common genetic disorder in the US. About 100,000 Americans are thought to be living with sickle cell disease, and each year another 1,000 babies are born with it. The majority of patients are black (about 60 to 80 percent in total), but it can affect other races, including people of Indian and Middle Eastern descent.

There are three main types of sickle cell disease: sickle cell anemia, SC, and SS. Each of these can also be mixed with other blood disorders, such as beta-thalassemia, which creates variations on each. The one people usually have heard of is sickle cell anemia. Mine is a very specific type called sickle-thal with arthritis, which is sickle cell type SC mixed with arthritis and beta-thalassemia, a blood disorder that reduces the production of hemoglobin, the protein in red blood cells that carries oxygen. I didn't receive a correct diagnosis until I was 28 years old, which has always caused problems because doctors have never known how to help me.

When you have sickle cell, your red blood cells get stuck on their way around your veins, causing blockages and stopping the oxygen from getting to your vital organs. Where there's a lack of oxygen, you can go into a crisis, an attack of severe pain, sometimes located only in a certain spot and sometimes all over your body. Often, it's hard to breathe or walk or even do something as basic as holding a pen. A crisis can happen without any warning. Just, bam! You're in the hospital again. If you go swimming, get on a plane, get caught in the rain, or experience a change in climate, you could fall ill. Even if I get really emotional or stressed out, a crisis can come on. Drinking alcohol thins your blood, as does flying on a plane, so that's a no-no, too. You don't always have to go to the hospital for a crisis, but if you can't get it under control at home right away, it usually lands you in a hospital bed. And, of course, I picked a career that is a real no-no for sickle cell patients because I'm always active, always traveling, and always on planes and in different climates.

Sickle cell disease currently does not have a cure, although they have found ways of curing unborn children and, in some rare cases, patients under the age of 40. That's the general cutoff because trying to cure someone as they get older, in most cases, can do more harm than good. That means there's no cure for me—at least right now. It's a lifelong disease and you have to manage it every single day. It's a learning process, too. What can your body handle? What's the breaking point? Each new experience, each new day, gives you a little more data on how to better survive. You figure out what works and what doesn't, and then you move forward from there. And you're always trying to figure out more because your body changes over time, and you'd be surprised how much doctors don't know and don't help. And honestly, some just don't care.

You'd think I'd have it all figured out by now. But, if I'm telling the truth, it's incredibly hard to live with this disease. It's incredibly hard to live with any disease. With sickle cell, you don't always know when a crisis is coming. One can arise at any time, in any place, totally debilitating you. Some days I wake up consumed by pain, which seems to manifest itself slightly differently every time. It's like knives stabbing me over and over again in my joints. The invisible knives leave no place untouched except my fingers and toes. It's impossible to function like that. Sometimes I can't even hold a glass of water. Usually, when I'm in a lot of pain, I can't walk. It hurts to lie down, but it hurts to sit up. Every breath I take throbs and each gasp of air comes in with a sharp twinge. I used to hate for my mom to carry me to the bathroom when I was sick as a kid, so I'd crawl there on all fours, no matter how much it hurt or how long it took. I was stubborn that way.

When you're strong and have a high tolerance for pain like me and you don't always act sick, you can go to the hospital in a crisis and sometimes the nurses will say, "Well, it doesn't look like anything's wrong." They don't always want to help you if you're not screaming and crying and acting a fool. But my mom taught me to calm down. When you scream or move around or get agitated, the pain gets worse. So if you mentally try to stabilize yourself, it can help. Sometimes people think I have a hard exterior or that I'm putting on a face, but it's not like that. When you have something so debilitating and so painful, you train yourself to stand strong and not complain and not look for any pity.

Maybe you can't fathom what it's like to feel the things I've felt—and that's been true of people around me a lot—but I bet you can imagine why strength through anything tough is so important. It's especially important if you have kids and they're in the hospital with you. You don't want your kids to know you think you might die. And there were some instances where I really could have died. I don't want my daughter or my son to feel my pain. I've felt like I'm dying inside and I've had to keep a normal face on. It's a double-edged sword, because I am afraid and I do need support, but I also understand that my own strength is essential, both for me and for those around me.

It can be especially scary because, as I've learned, a lot of doctors don't know much about it. That's true about most doctors when it comes to a lot of things, but they don't want to admit it because it's their job to know. Medicine is technically a science, but I've found much of it is actually just guesswork. They'll stick a needle in you or give you a drug even if they're not sure what it's going to do. They treat the symptoms, not the cause. I've been very mistreated in hospitals over the years. A good doctor looks at the whole person, not just the disease. They learn your name, and they ask how you're doing and find out your medical history. Good nurses do the same. They show kindness and they treat you like a person, not an object.

But when you spend as much time as I have in a hospital bed, you learn that some doctors and some nurses are not caring at all. When I was a child, during one particular hospital stay, I remember feeling really sick and not wanting to eat. My mama left to go to the lobby for 10 minutes and the nurse took it upon herself to force-feed me. She stood over me, a bite of liver in her hand.

"No," I shook my head. "No, thank you." Instead of listening to me, she pressed my mouth open and shoved the food into my throat. When my mom returned, she was furious. The nurse was fired for it, and to this day, I can't stand liver.

I was turned from a patient into a guinea pig, especially when I was young. Doctors gave me all sorts of conflicting drugs, and I've been given drugs that constipate me and then drugs that act as a laxative. They've given me drugs that have made me break out, throw up, scratch my skin uncontrollably, and hallucinate; some almost stopped my heart. They loaded me with really powerful painkillers, which has been a nightmare. It's put my body through so much. Sometimes I feel like the medication has done more harm than good.

There are three types of medication that work best for sickle cell to contain the pain. The strongest are Demerol, Dilaudid, and morphine. They administer them through a pump in your IV, usually every 15 minutes in little spurts, or through your actual IV every 4 to 6 hours. I itch on all three of them, because my body rejects pain medicine. Dilaudid has made me puke so hard that one of my ribs cracked, and it has almost stopped my heart and almost killed me, so it's not an option. I'm allergic to morphine, which makes it pretty miserable. I see rats every time I take it, so they switched me over to Demerol. But after Michael Jackson died, that was taken off the market. It's a really dangerous drug. It's given people seizures and halted their heart from beating. So now I'm back on morphine when I'm in the hospital, and I have to deal with all the crazy side effects. The doctors give me Benadryl and something for my stomach so I won't puke before taking the morphine. It's a rock and a hard place—the pain from the disease or the misery of the drugs that are supposed to help you.

Because I've been given so many drugs in the hospital and had so many IVs, my veins are pretty burned out. The worst part is when they take you off the medication because you go through withdrawal. It's important to wind down slowly, so they lower the dosage gradually. You have to deal with hot and cold flashes, shaking, crazy dreams, bad nerves—it's the worst. Your body has to sweat out all the super-strong drugs you didn't even want in the first place. It can be really traumatic, even though you get used to the process.

I have all this knowledge now, but no one knew anything in the '70s when I was growing up—or in the '80s or '90s, for that matter. When I was a baby I cried all the time. No one could figure out why, and there wasn't a lot of research available on genetic disorders like sickle cell back then. But my mom knew something wasn't right. My early years were spent packing and unpacking a suitcase to go to the hospital in Des Moines. Even though we didn't understand what my disease was yet, we got to know the signs of the sickness coming on. The pain would weave through my limbs and I'd cry and cry.

Sometimes I'd get delirious and not know where I was. Other times my face would swell up really badly and I'd get super pale with pink lips and dark circles under my eyes.

My mom was there by my side the whole time, comforting me and holding my hand. She used to sing a melody using my name to calm me down. "I know a girl, a pretty lil' girl, oh, Tionne, oh, Tionne Tenese," my mama would croon. And it helped. She took me to get a special treat on the way to the hospital every time. Sometimes we went for sugar biscuits at Mustard's, or to Smitty's Donuts, or to Tasty Tacos. The food would make me forget about the pain and the fear, and for a few moments, the tears would ebb.

There were a lot of things that could bring on a crisis when I was a kid. By trial and error my mom figured out some of them: too much heat dehydrated me, and too much cold made me achy and my bones hold on to the low temperature. Swimming in a chilly pool or the ocean, drinking milk, playing in the snow, or getting something out of the freezer could all trigger a crisis. Stress, exhaustion, and fighting all messed me up, too. It felt like anything and everything could be a trigger.

In 1977, after years of illness and uncertainty, my mom took me back to Mercy Hospital in Des Moines. An Indian doctor, whose name I don't remember, did a few tests. They'd been testing me since I was born, trying to figure out why I was always getting sick, but this time the doctor claimed to have found the reason.

"She has sickle cell anemia and allegetic arthritis," he told my mom while I sat on the table. "It's serious."

"What does that mean?" my mom asked. I leaned forward. I wanted to know, too. Maybe he could get rid of all my pain.

"She won't live past 30," he explained, bluntly. "She can't ever have children. She's going to be disabled her entire life."

I was only 7 years old, but I wasn't too young to understand what he was saying. I looked around the room, staring at my mama and this doctor. Who was he talking about? This wasn't my story. I was going to be a famous performer. He was clearly mistaken.

My mom saw my confusion. She put her hand on my arm and lowered herself to look into my eyes. "Don't worry, honey," she said confidently. "God has the last say-so in your life."

That guy was the first doctor to be totally wrong, but certainly not the last. I knew better than to believe him, though. I was meant for something much bigger and much greater. I wasn't going to be the victim of a disease he didn't seem to know much about. I was going to be a star and no illness was going to get in my way.

Having this disease doesn't have to be a death sentence, although you can die from it. It doesn't mean your life can't be well-lived and happy. I'm proof of that. Ever since I came clean to the public that I have sickle cell disease in the mid-'90s, I've worked really hard to be an outspoken advocate for other sick people, especially kids. Doctors and medicine have come a long way since I was born, but there are still misconceptions about sickle cell. It's not always an easy life, although some people on the outside might think so because I have a strong persona. But it's possible to face those hard times head-on and survive.

This takes me to the other half of my story, which involves a very different version of the word *sick*. In TLC, I saw things and went places that most people can only dream of. TLC has released four albums since we formed in Atlanta, and we spent 2016 and 2017 making our fifth. We've had major successes and major struggles. There's been birth, death, bankruptcy, feuds, and, most important, relatable songs and timeless music. So many times I've heard our song "Waterfalls" being played in a store or on a TV show or from a car window while I'm driving down the street or standing in an elevator. As I was suffering from the pain of sickle cell disease and as I was grappling to figure out how to live with it, I didn't feel like I had to be defined by my illness. I'm a performer first, and I just happen to have a lifelong problem to deal with. Some of the most important moments of my life have arrived because of TLC.

Here are some examples of that. The two people who had the most musical influence on me were Michael Jackson and Prince. Throughout our career, I met both, which was seriously insane. I can still barely believe it. I even got to work with Michael Jackson when TLC performed at two of his Heal the World benefit shows, which was a dream come true. In 2000, TLC performed at Madison Square Garden, the holy grail of venues. It was sold out, which is a really big deal. During the show, we launched into our single "No Scrubs." Suddenly, through the speakers came the twang of a guitar. It wasn't one of our band's guitars, but something about it sounded familiar. I turned around and it was Prince. I'd met him before that night, but I never imagined that he'd come up onstage with us. The reverberation of his guitar strings echoed around me and out into the crowd, urging a cheer from the audience, who were just as surprised as we were.

In that moment, I almost stopped singing. All I could think was, "This is not happening to me." I forgot, for a moment, that I was T-Boz. I temporarily lost the knowledge that I was supposed to be a celebrity, too. I went into fan mode. I wasn't Tionne on this stage, so I couldn't get star-struck. I had to consciously breathe and remind myself to keep singing. I had to silently tell myself to get it together. And even though he was onstage with all of us, I felt like he was there with just me. At the end of the song, Prince just vanished. We kept performing. We didn't even get a chance to speak to him after the show—he arrived and then disappeared, like a magician fading in and out of the room.

As you'll see, the journey of TLC is an incredible one. I believe everything happens for a reason, and it seems like a lot of things lined up for us to become what we became. There are stories of rebellion, of delight, of triumph. We set out to be trendsetters and we did just that. We've toured the world, playing on massive stages in huge rooms to crowds of thousands. We've won awards and become a household name. Our fans from the '90s have had children and have brought those children to our recent shows, making us a band for multiple generations. We were able to do it because we worked hard, cared a lot, and believed it was possible.

The music industry can be hard, too. TLC learned that early on. We lost a lot of money. The music business is exactly that—a business. You get to make meaningful art, but at the end of the day it's about the bottom line. I signed my name to a contract at 19 years old that I was stuck to for years against my will. I was subservient to what other people thought was best for me and for TLC. People in this industry want to exploit you and exploit your talent, and you have to learn not to let them. I almost threw in the towel on music more than once. TLC had great successes, but we also had some failures, too. And worst of all, we lost one of our own, a tragedy that lingers with me to this day.

I'm a person who is afflicted with disease. Sickle cell hasn't been the only health scare I've dealt with. But the slang version of the word *sick* means something else, "awesome" or "excellent." My life, as hard as some of it has been, has been incredible. I wouldn't trade it for the world. So to say I've had a sick life is twofold: I've been in and out of the hospitals, but my life has also been awesome. I have these two stories converging into one, where sometimes I'm Tionne and sometimes I'm T-Boz.

But the truth is that both of these women are the same person. We're both mothers, daughters, sisters, friends, artists, and survivors. We both know that it takes hard work to succeed and that giving up is never an option. We also both know that after the darkness there is always light. It can be hard to see in the moment when you feel trapped and blinded, but it's there, waiting to shine in. You have to have faith that the light will come. When I'm sick, I always take myself to a peaceful place. I love water, so I imagine a cave of three waterfalls and a stream that takes you to a beautiful beach. It's calm and quiet, and it helps me remember that everything will be okay.

I was given a death sentence of 30 years old. I lived past it. I was given another death sentence, by another doctor, of 45 years old. I lived past that one, too. I was never supposed to have children, and my daughter Chase is now a teenager. I recently adopted a son from birth named Chance. I was told I'd be disabled my entire life, but I still get onstage and perform my heart out every month. So no one can tell you what you're going to be. Only you and God know your path, and like my mama said, he has the last say-so.

What makes you keep going when your body continually fails you? Why do you stand up again and again and keep trying to survive? For myself, it's for many reasons: for love, for my daughter, for my son, for my family, for music, for the fans. I've always kept standing back up, no matter what obstacle was placed in front of me, because that's the only thing you can do. And if I can do that, after all these years, anyone can. The truth is that anything you really want in life is never easy—but it's worth it.

When I was first starting out as a performer, before TLC blew up, I was working on my dance moves with my friend Devyne Stephens, who is a choreographer.

"Tionne," he asked, "do you know what a true choreographer is?"

"No," I said. "What is it?"

"It's not a person who learns a dance and teaches it to another," he told me. "It's a person who creates the dance and makes the world follow."

"Well, that's what I'm going to be," I confirmed. And I thought about it. I wanted to be a true choreographer. Someone who could create and make the world follow. When you're an artist, you want to be a trendsetter. Or, at least, the best artists do. I wanted to be successful like Michael Jackson or Prince, but still be known for being myself. I always want to reach for the top in everything I do, whether it's writing new music or creating a music video or even writing a book. I embraced that idea throughout TLC's career. I created the dances for some of our biggest hits, like "Waterfalls," "What about Your Friends," and "Creep." They became iconic. And like Devyne said, I got to watch the world do those dances. He really helped me with my confidence as a performer and as a dancer, and I saw the proof of my work linger with our fans.

When I was born, anything was possible. The world was limitless. But I struck out on my own path and chose my own way. I was wholly myself throughout all of it. I may not have always shared my stories with the public or opened the curtain completely, but I've never deviated from who I am as both Tionne and as T-Boz. That is the key. You should always be who you are. Just because none of the girls are wearing baggy pants and dancing with the guys doesn't mean you can't. Just because the music industry expects women to sex themselves up to sell music doesn't mean you have to. Just because the doctors tell you that you'll die doesn't mean you will. You get to choreograph your own life. And if you do that, if you make the moves your way, the world will follow.

CHAPTER 2

The MTB Thang

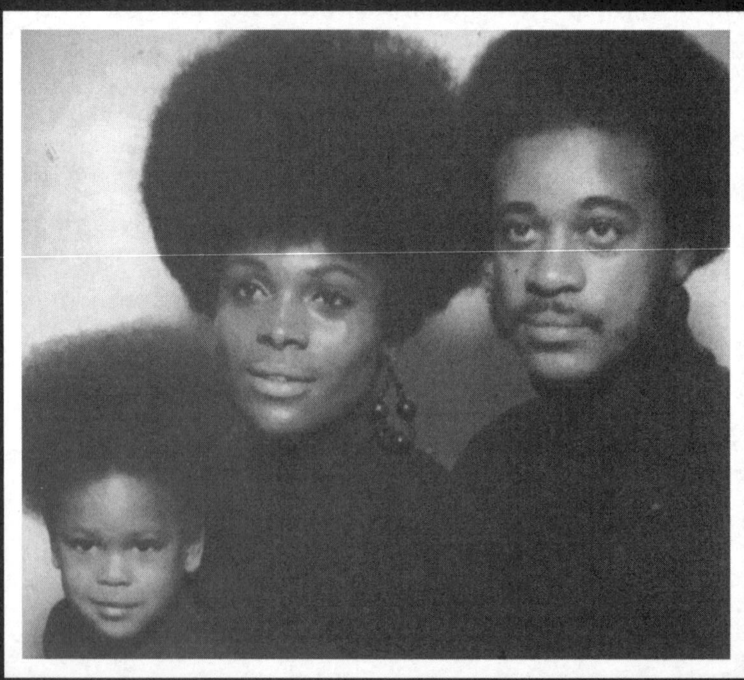

TLC has a saying. If something feels right, like it's destined for you, it's an "MTB thang." It means "meant to be." It's something you say about an inevitability or about fate. Throughout my life, since I was a little kid, I've been prone to premonitions. Sometimes I feel when things are going to happen. I certainly can't predict everything, but often, in your gut, you know when it's MTB. For me, performing was one of those things. I was born to sing and dance, and there was never going to be another path for me.

That became clearer and clearer as I grew up, even if I wasn't always certain exactly what that life would look like.

The first time I went on a stage I was 7. My mom entered me in a pageant called Little Miss Black Des Moines. I was a black kid growing up in a predominately white neighborhood in Iowa. We lived in a medium-sized house that my mama still owns today. I was a natural performer, always dancing and trying to play some instrument, and this was going to be my grand entrance. They thought it would be good for me to perform a skit for the pageant, but I refused to rehearse in front of anyone, even my mama. She had a friend who was an acting coach and helped me, and I practiced a lot. I was a little skeptical about doing a pageant and I felt nervous, but still I wanted to win. The funny thing is that I will dance and sing in front of anyone, but speaking before a crowd is hard for me. I don't like people staring—which is true to this day.

The pageant was held every year, and this year's program had a cartoon sketch of a little black Shirley Temple girl with curly hair on the cover. I don't think I really wanted to do it, but I had committed and wanted to keep my word. I also really did want to win! I wore a beanie hat just like Rerun on *What's Happening!!*, and I went onstage and did my little skit. As I look back now, it seems strange that I didn't sing or dance. But it was my first time performing for a big audience and I wasn't sure exactly what I wanted to be yet. I loved being in the spotlight, all the parents watching me and clapping. I was a star, if only for a few minutes.

I didn't win. The girl who got first place played an instrument—I can't remember which one. The judges sat on the side of the stage, so they couldn't see how her legs were cocked open the whole time she played. Everyone in the crowd could see her panties. So she beat me and I came in second place. But I know if they had seen her underwear, I would have come in first.

I knew from then on that I wanted to be a performer. I sang at the Maple Street Baptist Church every weekend with my mama. She was like the Patti LaBelle of the church, the big kahuna. I always looked up to her. Her song was "I'm Going Over Yonder" and mine was "Sinner You're Gonna Be Sorry." Since my mom was the main star, everyone called me "Little Gayle." Everyone would urge me to sing, saying, "Go ahead, Little Gayle." But I wanted to be myself. I would think to myself, "Stop calling me my mama's name. I am not my mama. I'm 'bout to be on TV. I'm 'bout to blow up." I was Tionne, not Little Gayle. And don't get me wrong—I looked up to my mama. Like any little girl, I wanted to be just like her. But I still knew I wanted to make a name for myself.

I didn't perform outside of church when I was younger, but I wanted to learn new things. "I wanna do this," I'd tell my mama about something. And then a few days later, "I don't wanna do this anymore." But she let me try it all so I could figure out what I liked. I tried tae kwon do, but after the second day, that was it for me. I didn't like it. Then my mom paid for me to take 2 weeks of piano classes. After those 2 weeks I announced, "I don't think this is what I want to do either." She said, "Tionne, nobody has time to pay for you to start something you don't finish."

I assured her that if I took up dance classes I would not quit. So when I was 12, she found a program at the local rec center and enrolled me. I breezed through those classes like jazz and modern dance. They kept moving me up to more advanced classes. Within a few weeks, they put me in the adult intermediate class and offered to let me perform in this big show. I danced to "Wade in the Water," clad in this African outfit and no shoes. Just me, one other kid, and a bunch of adults. After that there was nowhere to advance up to. I was done with the dance classes.

I started realizing that I might have real talent. That kind of praise helped me understand that I had something special. I didn't know I could dance as well as I did because usually it was just my cousins saying, "Ask Tionne, she can dance." I loved Michael Jackson, so I practiced the moves to "Billie Jean" every single day religiously. I worked on those moves way harder than I worked on homework. We had this mirrored table in our basement, and I used it to put on Prince concerts for my friends after school. They were crazy enough to actually sit there and watch me. Dancing, for me, felt easy and natural. My mom can dance, so I don't get it from nowhere. I think maybe it came in my DNA.

I learned a lot from my mama. She taught me how to hustle. We lived in a big house on a nice street, but sometimes we were broke. We sold whatever T-shirts were currently popular on the street corner and at swap meets, and dug through the couch cushions for change when we needed money. I don't know where the shirts came from, but I think my mama bought them in bulk. We even sold car wax and necklace charms dipped in gold leaf. Sometimes we ate watermelon and popcorn for dinner. But my clothes were always nice and they were always clean. I was taught to present myself well no matter the circumstances.

It was important that I had my mom because my dad was inconsistent and a habitual liar. He was a musician when I was a kid and now he's a pastor, of sorts. I like to joke and call him Reverend Do Wrong. When I was a young kid, my parents' marriage started to break apart. My dad never kept his promises. When I was 5, he called on Christmas Eve and said, "Hey, T-Booger, come wait by the window and I'll bring your gifts." I sat by that window all night long and he didn't come. When my mom tried to put me to bed, I screamed, "No, my daddy is coming." I finally fell asleep on the couch. I woke up in my bed on Christmas morning, and my mom made sure I had the best Christmas without him. She moved out all the living room furniture and got me a little merry-go-round and a big toy roller coaster you could ride on. It took my mind off my dad for a little while.

My father was a bigamist and cheated on my mom when they were still together. My mom found out later that he didn't show that Christmas because he was getting married to someone else. So I don't know why he told me to wait for him by that window. When I was growing up, my mama didn't believe in running men in and out of the house. She raised me to be a strong, independent woman. Men could come second, or not at all. She knew not to rely on anyone else but herself, especially after how badly my daddy treated her. My mama did everything herself.

"Tionne," she'd tell me. "It's your job to make sure your kids are protected. It's your job to make sure a child is straight. Remember that when you grow up and start a family."

I saw my dad on and off as I was growing up. He was in a band and they toured around a lot. He was out in the world spreading his love, if you know what I mean. When I was really young, before my parents broke up, he asked my cousin Ronnie, who was 17, to come along to Florida with his band. "Don't go," I begged Ronnie. I felt like something bad was going to happen. "I have a feeling. Don't leave." But he went. A week later we found out that my dad's bandmate Delbert had murdered Ronnie. He stabbed him in the chest with a butcher knife in a dispute over some money.

It was my first real brush with death. It hit me really hard. Because my dad was never around, Ronnie felt like the man in my life. He was the only grown-up big guy I knew. He played with me and we'd watch TV together. I was furious that my dad took him away from me. It didn't make sense. I didn't understand why I kept losing all the significant men in my life. I was so sad, and I was still young, so death was harder to wrap my head around. I knew about death, but I hadn't known it would feel so permanent. Ronnie was just gone.

To this day, my biggest pet peeve is someone not keeping their word. It always reminds me of my father. If you tell me one lie, I'll never trust you again.

My issues with my dad lingered a little heavier after that. I didn't feel like he had my back. He let his girlfriend—who later became his wife (and who we will call Bertildia)—abuse me and barely noticed. I think some women have an issue with another woman's child, so I was a problem for her to begin with. Bertildia would knock my food on the floor at McDonald's and would bat my hand away if I wanted to grab my dad's hand or just take his hand if I was already holding it, and he'd do nothing. She braided my hair too tight, which you can't do because it gives you bumps and it's really painful. You can lose your hair from too much tension. One night, while I was visiting them in Florida, she tried to force me into a scalding hot bath that would have hurt my skin. I ran out, called my mom, and said, "Bertildia is trying to burn me." My mom hung up, grabbed her purse, and drove straight to the airport. It felt like only minutes had passed when I heard the door fly open, hinges creaking.

"Where the fuck she at?" my mama hollered. She packed up my stuff and we went home. My dad hid Bertildia, which was probably for the best.

Another time, my mom and I flew to Florida and my dad was supposed to come meet us at the airport. He never showed up. He hadn't seen me in a while, but he couldn't be bothered to come. I had to talk to a psychiatrist after that happened. I started poking my dolls' eyes out because I was so mad that he left us at the airport.

Dads can make or break you as a kid; my issues with him have continued throughout my life. When I first met my dad's second wife—we can call her Helda—I reached my hand out in greeting and she folded her arms as if I was diseased. She simply said, with spite, "Where's the bathroom?" I thought to myself, *Oh boy, here we go again!* Helda tried to entice two of my boyfriends and later my husband by showing them her panties. She tried to invite herself on my husband's tour bus by telling him she gave good head. I've never been trying to live out a real-life *Jerry Springer* episode, but my dad has made that difficult.

My mom did her best during all this drama with my dad. She stood by me and gave me endless amounts of love. But, no matter what, she couldn't pay me to believe my dad loved me. She worried because I was constantly sick and she didn't always know how to help me. I'm sure it must have been awful to see me in pain. She held my hand and smiled and sang as we dealt with health scare after health scare. I only saw my dad in the hospital when my parents were still together. Once they broke up, I didn't get any more visits from him for the rest of my childhood! I guess it was because he lived out of state. In my adult years I remember some visits—if he happened to be in town—but I can't recall him ever flying out to see me when I was sick.

I want to be clear about something: I don't dislike my dad. The Bible says "Love thy father," and that's important. Even though I felt like he wronged me early on, I still love him. Today, we're trying to build a better relationship, and we speak from time to time, mostly through text messaging. I know now that having issues with my dad is where a lot of my anger came from early on in my life. I was mad that he used to lie to me and it turned out that the world wasn't this perfect little place I thought it should be. I wanted things to be different, so I was mad about that a lot.

I finally figured out that all of these issues with my dad also resulted in me choosing the wrong men. I was looking for the protective vibe that he didn't give me. Your dad is supposed to protect you, but for me it was always my mom instead. I didn't look as closely at men as I should have. I just looked at whether they could protect me. I didn't bother to consider the intricate details that build a relationship. I made the wrong choices. That was a real life lesson.

When I think about my dad, I realize how far I've come since those early years. Here's what I know now about anger: No matter who the person is or the situation, you only hurt yourself more if you hold a grudge. It's not healthy. That person just continues on with their life, and you're the one who's hurt and left behind damaging yourself. They won't change. So you have to learn to just get over it. Let it go and learn to heal. Don't get stuck in the past. My dad has changed some, but he's never admitted to some of his lies. My anger didn't change anything for me. I know that now. It actually made a lot of things worse.

But back then, as my health became more and more of an issue, I always had my mom by my side. I've said it before and I'll say it again: My mom was the best possible example of a parent. She showed me enough love for both of them, especially when I was sick.

It was always a learning process on how to deal with the illness. It was scary to discover as a young child that I was different, that I had to grapple with something other people didn't. I couldn't go swimming. Other kids could have ice cream and I wasn't allowed to have cow's milk. I drank baby formula for a long time because it was the only option besides actual milk, and I got teased for it. I was in and out of the hospital a lot. I knew doctors and nurses by name. Once I was in the newspaper because I spent so much time in the children's wing. The fact that I was sick was part of my reality, but as time passed, regardless of how ill I felt, it became something of a second nature. Mostly, I was more interested in singing and dancing than I was in worrying about my health.

We moved around somewhat when I was young, trying to find a place to call home. My mom was a get-up-and-go kind of woman, and she didn't have my dad to tie her down. So if she wanted to do something, she did it. She grew tired of the Midwest, and I think the South seemed like an awesome place to her. Her first choice was Houston, although I'm not entirely sure why. She closed the Montessori school she owned and we headed south, renting out our house in Des Moines. We lived there for 9 months, in a two-bedroom apartment that felt so much smaller to me than our three-story house in Des Moines, and those months were filled with bad luck. It was not MTB.

Mom worked three jobs in preparation for the move to Houston. She hired a moving company to haul all our stuff from Des Moines to Houston, and I watched them load it all into a trailer and drive away. Two days later the phone rang. The truck had been vandalized and burned by the movers on the way to Houston. My mama hustled me into the car and drove in a fury to see what was left. When we arrived, finally, the trailer and everything left in it was a smoldering mess. Almost nothing was left. The movers had taken most of our lives with them—the TV, the stereo, the nicest pieces of furniture, and all our pictures and memories. And then, apparently, they lit the rest on fire. I stood there, next to my mama, and stared at the ashes. All we had left were some suitcases of clothes in the trunk of our car. There was a sad look on my mom's face and I didn't know how to comfort her.

But we knew we had to start again and that we had each other. My mom did her best to fill our new apartment and to make me feel like it was home. I felt like a happy, normal kid most of the time. I liked everything about Houston except for the time I was chased by a big, scary German shepherd. I had a bad history with dogs that started with my dad's dog Kipper, who bit my right eye, lip, and stomach. Thanks to him, I've always had a fear of dogs. And, I'll admit, I had another childhood phobia I developed when I stayed over at a friend's house in the projects. I loved eating Raisin Bran, just like my mama ate, and my friend's parents told me to make myself at home. I climbed on the counter to get a bowl and my knee knocked over the cereal box. Raisins ran everywhere. And they kept running. It turned out they weren't raisins, they were roaches. So to this day I can't have raisins.

In Houston, the bad luck continued. Soon after we settled in, someone hit our little Volkswagen and totaled it. So we had no furniture and no car. I kept getting sick, too. My illness would flare up and I'd feel tired or achy and I'd go to the hospital. It was a stressful time.

It got worse. My mom used to help out this young guy named Vincent, who she was really kind to. We met him in Houston, and she took to him and always did good by him. My mama has a habit of taking in strays, and that's what she did with him. One day she put me in our car and we drove over to an apartment.

"Stay here," she told me. I watched through the window as she marched upstairs, dragged Vincent out of the apartment and back down the stairs, and beat his ass. She got back in the car.

"What did he do?" I asked.

"He stole your college money," she replied. "I've been saving Susan B. Anthony coins since you were born, and he used the money to buy drugs. It's gone."

After that, my mom had enough of Houston. She was worried about my safety because a 3-year-old kid had her throat slit just around the corner from our apartment. One day when she was a few minutes late picking me up from school, my mama arrived to find a man trying to lure me into his car. Another time we came home and found the maintenance man walking out of our house. That was the end of Texas for us.

We spent 6 months in California after that so my mama could take care of my aunt Wanda after her surgery, and then, when I was 9, it was decided that we'd move to Atlanta. My mama didn't know anyone there, but she said it seemed like the right place to start over. I think she was inspired by the Gladys Knight & the Pips song "Midnight Train to Georgia." She used to sing it all the time. When we arrived we still didn't have a lot of furniture. Our first apartment there, in Union City, was filled with boxes. For Thanksgiving, my mama, her best friend Una Mae, and Una Mae's daughter Tae Tae (who I considered my aunt and cousin) covered some of the boxes with a cloth and served dinner on it like a table. It felt like home, suddenly. I started to feel like I belonged there. Having Una and Tae Tae there helped a lot.

I missed Iowa—I'd been dragged out of Des Moines kicking and screaming at first—but I felt a connection to Atlanta.

I liked the vibe and the music. Everything felt new and current. The weather, which was so much warmer and temperate than the Midwest, was somewhat better for my health. My body reacts badly to the cold, and I always ached when we were in Des Moines. Of course, sometimes it's bad for me to get too hot, too, because I get sick or dehydrated, but it was better overall. I felt good and things felt exciting.

After 3 years in Atlanta, we moved back to Des Moines. It felt like a blessing and a curse to me. My mama got pregnant, and she wanted us to move in with my grandma, Velma, so she could have some help and so my brother could be born in Iowa like me. We packed up again and headed back to the Midwest. I didn't realize I'd be so jealous when Koko came home from the hospital. (His real name is Carnoy but we called him Koko as a child. He is now called Kayo.) Everyone kept coming over to the house and fawning over him. I didn't like sharing the attention.

"Mama," I said one day, "when is Koko going back?"

"What do you mean?" she asked.

"When's he going back to the hospital?" I said.

"He's not," she said. "He's here to stay."

So I had to come around to him, even if I didn't like it at first. And soon enough I loved him and I was proud to be his sister.

My mama thought it was important for me to know how to cook. When I was 12, she taught me to prepare full-course meals, and I'd make dinner while she was working at UPS. She worked long hours, so I was responsible for making Koko dinner and helping him with his homework while he was growing up. I felt like his second mom, and our connection got closer and closer over the years. Now we have companies and work in the music industry together. He produced a lot on our latest album.

In Des Moines, I loved living with my grandma. I admired her so much and she was so sweet and wise. I loved going with her to Native American powwows to learn about our heritage. She took me to see the Commodores, my first concert ever. In the afternoon, she watched soap operas—*The Young and the Restless, As the World Turns, Guiding Light*—and every day I sat right beside her. We gossiped during the commercial breaks, and she'd explain what was going on in the soaps. She knew every detail of the characters and the plot. She loved black coffee, which I didn't understand. She made me a special milk drink out of Coffee-mate creamer since I couldn't have milk.

My mom always planned to move back to Atlanta after having Koko, so we didn't stay in Des Moines permanently. She went to Atlanta to find us a new place to live and look for a job, leaving me with my grandma—which, obviously, was something I was very into. I lived with Grandma for a month, and every morning she'd get up and make me a big breakfast. I always helped her clean up the kitchen afterward. We didn't always agree on food, though.

"Tionne," she said one day, "try this." It was a peanut butter, jelly, and banana sandwich. Ew. But I loved my grandma so I took a small, tentative bite. It was so mushy. The ingredients didn't belong together at all.

"Grandma," I said, still chewing, "sorry, but that is nasty. I don't know how you eat it."

"Tionne, food is not nasty," she replied. She was very serious. She felt that parents worked hard to feed their kids, so you should eat everything you were given and be thankful.

My family was really important to me when I was growing up and they still are. I spent a lot of time with my cousins and my aunts Ressie, Velva, and Wanda. My uncle Quynton and I were close when I was younger, but I was especially close with my uncle Victor. He's the reason I have a complex about feet. He had these crusty feet, and he would hold me down and rub his feet on my face. The dry skin would roll down my cheeks. He told me, "You have to learn how to get out from under my hold." I learned how to wiggle out from under people's legs and put them in a choke hold. I have a lifelong complex about feet thanks to him, but I also learned how to get myself out of compromising situations, which helped me later on.

I was a family-oriented kid, but that doesn't mean that my teenage years were a breeze. Once I got to high school, I started getting into trouble. I was a nice girl, but I loved street folks. I always wanted to hang with them because I thought they were so cool and real. I stole clothes from Macy's and from Rich's, which I learned from my friend from New York. If you heisted something from Rich's and it was under $50, you could return it for cash. You didn't need the receipt if it was under $50. At Macy's, for anything over $100 they'd send you a check in the mail if you returned it. My friends and I had the whole system worked out, and we never got caught. My mom didn't know, but she knew I was up to dicey stuff. She knew she raised me better than that. But if she told me not to do something, chances were that I still might try it (depending on how badly I wanted it).

One weekend when I was 16, my mom went out of town and my aunt Velva was in charge of watching me. Before Velva left for work for the day she said, "Tionne, do not drive the car. Your mom parked it in a certain way. She'll know if you moved it." But I was smarter than that. I took a piece of chalk and marked around the wheels so I could put it back the same way. Me and my friend Lil' Kim (not the famous rapper) got in the car, I backed it out of the driveway, and we took off for the Greenbriar Mall to steal some clothes so I could look fly to dance at the skating rink on Sunday. My aunt wasn't going to be back until after 4:00 p.m., so I knew we had mad time to spare. Enough time to hit up Blimpie on the way home. I had it all figured out: 10 minutes at Blimpie, 10 minutes to drive home, 10 minutes for the car to cool down.

Except the car wouldn't start. We were sitting in the Blimpie parking lot, thinking, "Aw, junk!" I begged everyone who came by for a jump start. Finally, with only 20 minutes to spare, some guy jumped the car and we leapt in and gunned it, heading back to my house. I went straight through a stoplight as this white guy zoomed and revved around the corner. I tapped the back of his car. Oh, no. Even though it was his fault for pulling in front of me, I took off. I just kept going and he started chasing us.

"You fuckin' niggers," he shouted at us. "Imma fuckin' kill you, you fuckin' niggers!"

Kim and I started crying. "Oh my god," I screamed. "He's racist. He's gonna kill us!" I knew it was serious once he used the n-word since we were in the South, where the KKK dwell.

I kept my foot on the gas, careening down the road. I turned and sped, trying to figure out the way back to my house, tears pouring down my face. I was lost and so afraid. I flew through a cul-de-sac and somehow got my bearings. The guy chasing us got stuck, and we lost him around the corner. With minutes to spare, I pulled the car back into the driveway, lining it up with the chalk lines. Kim and I frantically tried to rub the chalk off the pavement as we straightened our clothes and wiped away our tears.

By the time my aunt came home, shortly after, Kim and I were sitting in the living room, pretending nothing had happened. We were calm by then.

"Tionne," my aunt Velva said. "I know you stole the car. The hood is hot." My heart sank. After all that, I still got caught.

"Please don't tell my mama!" I begged. I got away with it, barely. But it was a good thing that guy never figured out who hit his car or followed us home. My aunt Velva didn't tell my mama. She knew there'd be hell to pay if she told. And, thankfully, there were no dents as evidence.

During my teens, I had a boyfriend for several years. I don't need to reveal his real name, so let's call him Calvin. He was one of those street people I loved hanging out with. I lost my virginity to him, and we stayed together a long time. He got me into some bad things. When I was 17, he got me messed up in this check scam. I had a checking account, so one day he asked me to cash a check for him. It was for a few thousand bucks—not that much. I didn't think anything of it. What I didn't know was that the checks had been stolen from a major corporation in another state. His buddy stole hundreds of thousands of dollars by writing big checks and cashing them. Calvin wrote only a couple of the checks, but he was affiliated with this other guy.

At the time, my mom was working for UPS. She made good money, and we had big-screen TVs and nice furniture. She'd worked really hard to give my brother and me a nice home. A few days after I cashed the check for Calvin, I came home and the phone rang. It was one of the neighbors.

"We see people hanging in the trees looking at your house," he said. "Look outside."

What? Suddenly everything went into high gear. It was like an action movie. Guys from the FBI kicked in the door and busted through the windows. They were everywhere. They started to trash the house and dump drawers out. I had no idea what they were looking for.

The FBI guys had guns and were yelling, "Get on the ground!" My mom complied and looked at me. If looks could kill, that one would have. I would be dead. I got on the floor, too. My brother wasn't home—he was at his godmother's house—so it was just me and my furious mother trying to figure out why the FBI was here. And there was no reason why the FBI would show up at the house of an honest working woman unless her crazy-ass daughter who'd been hanging with the wrong people had done something bad.

The FBI questioned my mom for a long time. "How did you afford to buy this TV?" they asked. They acted like she was a criminal when all along it was me who had messed up. Ultimately, though, it came out why they were here. It was the checks. I got questioned next.

"I did it as a favor," I explained. "I gave them the money and didn't think anything of it." That was true—I didn't keep a dime.

The FBI made me go to the bank and write a confession letter explaining that I had nothing to do with it. I was facing years in jail if they convicted me for this. I could have been in really big trouble. They ended up arresting the guy who was leading the charge on the check scam, and they let me go. They decided I wasn't lying, which I wasn't, and that I had nothing to do with it, which I didn't. That guy got sent back to North Carolina or wherever he was from to face the charges. I still have my confession letter somewhere. It's hilarious to read now. Calvin and I stayed together for a while, although our relationship was really toxic. He went to jail later for something he didn't do, which seems ironic.

I got put on punishment by my mama, but it was nothing major because I knew how bad I'd screwed up. My mom simply said, "I don't want to talk to you right now because I might hurt you." She'd worked so hard for everything she had. I felt terrible. Some people do this kind of stuff while on drugs or while drunk, but I was of sound mind. I worked hard to get myself in order after that. I wanted to be the sort of daughter my mama was proud of. The things you learn from your parents when you're young are crucial. They lead by example. As I arrived at the end of high school, my path was ready to reveal itself. The stage was calling me. Even though I didn't have the term for it yet, things were really MTB.

CHAPTER 3

The TLC Tip

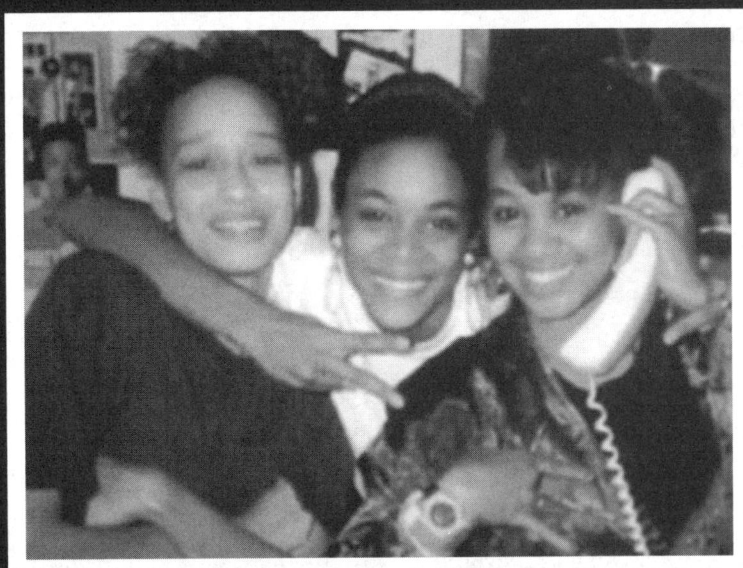

In the late '80s, all the kids hung out at a roller rink called Jelly Bean's. It was in Ben Hill, a neighborhood in southwestern Atlanta that, at the time, was considered the hood. Cars rolled up into the Jelly Bean's parking lot in squads. There was the Jetta crew, the Hyundai crew, the Jeep crew. Those cars were all that and then some, every single one painted up, fancy rims stuck on the wheels, and they looked cool even if they really weren't.

Later, you'd get the rich kids in their Porsches pulling in, sliding in between the cheap cars, and the motorcycle crew in after them. It was the place to be.

It cost 3 bucks to get inside, and I'd spend all week collecting those 3 dollars, begging quarters off people and hoarding the change. It felt like the end of the world if my mom said I couldn't go. I'd beg her to let me, whining and pleading like it was either this or death. If I misbehaved, my punishment was that I wasn't allowed to go to Jelly Bean's. "You're trippin',"

I'd mumble at my mama. "Why you gotta do that to me?"

But most weeks I went with my friend SaBrenna and we'd dress up like our lives depended on it. Baggy pants, colorful T-shirts, oversized sweatshirts, cool sneakers. I didn't have much money to buy new clothes, so she taught me how to shoplift. I stole whatever items I couldn't afford so I could have the latest trends. I had to look fresh, my hair had to look hella good, and I spent all week every week planning my outfit. It was a big deal to me. SaBrenna and I got there any way we could, usually hitching rides. We went almost every Sunday night for 3 years during high school.

Inside Jelly Bean's were guys with their trendy Gumby haircuts—like Bobby Brown in "Don't Be Cruel"—and girls in wildly bright clothes. There were drug dealers who had these ridiculously big phones inside even bigger phone cases sauntering around the rink, trying to impress everybody. Every week it was a fashion show, a talent show, and a party all at the same time. Dallas Austin, who later ended up being TLC's main producer and the father of Chilli's child, went there (and so did the guys from Outkast, although I didn't know them then). I knew Dallas and used to talk to him on the phone—long before I ever realized we'd work together. Some went to Jelly Bean's to hang out and to be seen. But others, like me, came to dance.

Every Sunday night some of the guys would gather on the dance floor (which was actually just the roller rink all cleared off) to battle. The room was packed, half the crowd cheering and half the crowd dancing across the floor. It was a real mob scene, everybody in, everybody grooving to the music, and trying to one up one another. It was only the guys who battled, but by the time I was a senior in high school I'd become

famous around town for my moves. I was the only girl they'd let in their dance crew—I danced the first time I ever went in there, people sweating all over the place—and I'd battle those dudes every single week.

I had all the popular moves: skipping, transforming, yeeking. When you were yeeking, a style of dance in Atlanta, you'd shout "Yeek!" as you did it. The battles were done with crews, but usually you faced off with someone solo in the center of the floor. You'd get in there, show your stuff, and the crowd would scream. Whoever got the loudest shouts was declared the winner. And you bet I won most of the rounds I battled.

Dancing was the thing I was best at, back then. School—not so much. I kept getting kicked out, and even though I was supposed to graduate from high school in 1988, I ended up being held back to the class of '89. I got kicked out of four high schools, much to my mama's dismay. She had to take me down to the Board of Education's office and convince them to find a school that would accept me. By the time she got me into one, I only had to go to the first 12 weeks of the year and then just wait for graduation to roll around. I took my graduation photos downtown all by myself because I'd messed up and hadn't been able to complete school with all my peers. I'd been kicked out of too many schools—and actually the whole school district—so I had to do the photos by myself. It seemed fitting that I'd have to get my pictures done solo. But I finished school. That's what mattered. It mattered to me and, more important, to my mama, who sat in the crowd while hundreds of kids got their diplomas before they arrived at the name "Watkins."

After high school, Mama wanted me to go to college. I

begged her to let me enroll in art school in New York City so I could study to be a fashion designer, but by the time she gave in, I'd decided I had other plans for my future. I wanted to stay in Atlanta, near my mama, so I took classes at a beauty school and specialized in doing nails. Not the career I wanted, but no 18-year-old girl knows what she really wants to do with her life. And at least this way I could make some money and pick my own hours. I didn't want someone bossing me around and telling me what to do and where to be. If you haven't already figured it out, I do not like authority figures. Not at all.

Toward the end of high school, while I was wasting time until graduation and spending every Sunday night at Jelly Bean's, I got a job at Lamonte's Beauty Supply, which was located in the Delowe Shopping Center in East Point. I ran the cash register, which I actually didn't hate, and the shop was owned by a guy who was rumored to be a big-time drug dealer. That meant we got paid in cash every 2 weeks, tax-free. Lamonte's was managed by Rico Wade, who gave me my first makeover and ended up being an important part of my career. It's hard to imagine now, but in my teens I dressed like a girl—way more than before my tomboy look kicked into full gear. One day we were at Rico's house and he handed me a pair of Girbaud jeans.

"What is this?" I asked.

"Put 'em on," he replied. My very first pair of baggy jeans. I tried them on right then. They were huge and fell around my ankles.

"They don't stay up," I said. "I don't understand how you make 'em stay up."

"Here," Rico said. He put a belt through the loops and

arranged the pants so they were dangling off my butt. "You look fly," he confirmed, nodding. It took a while for me to get used to those pants, but I did. From then on, I dressed like a boy. Rico called me the "brother with the lipstick" and the nickname stuck.

Rico knew a guy named Ian Burke, who was putting together a music group around Atlanta. Rico knew I could sing because I was always singing in the car and around him every day—and he definitely had seen me dance at Jelly Bean's—so he told Ian about me. At the time, Ian was managing a girl named Crystal Jones, who wanted to start a girl group. Rico had coincidentally also met Lisa, who'd recently moved to Atlanta from Philadelphia with almost nothing to her name. I didn't know Lisa at the time, but Ian asked both of us to come in and audition with Crystal. I didn't feel like going and had to work at the beauty salon where I'd recently become a hair apprentice, so I sent my friend Beverly in my place.

I didn't care. I wanted to be in a group, sure, but I wasn't about to spend my time running around town auditioning. So Rico made them come to me. He told Ian, "You have to see this girl. She's dope. Go to her house."

The next day Rico, Ian, and Crystal showed up at my mama's house. Lisa, who they'd accepted into the group the night before, waited in the car outside. I sang two songs, "That Girl" by Stevie Wonder and "Wanna Get with U" by Guy, and danced in the living room. I was in.

The first time I actually met Lisa was at Crystal's house, where we joined up to rehearse. Lisa had come to Atlanta with a keyboard, a few bucks, and a Honey Bun. She had this baby face with huge, pretty eyes. I liked her immediately. At the time, everyone called her QT, which was a perfect name because she was seriously adorable. Crystal introduced us.

"Hey, how you doin'?" I said.

"Hey, girl," she said.

And that was it. We hit it off. In that first moment, we just connected. And we connected on everything, period. After that, we'd sit on the floor of Crystal's house, talk about life, and laugh—a lot. Anything she would say, I'd laugh, and anything I'd say, she'd laugh. And Crystal just sat there like a third wheel. I sensed in those first few days that Lisa would become someone really important in my life, and she did. She was eventually my close friend and creative partner. We had this strong bond. I knew she was meant to become a special person in my life, somehow.

Our group with Crystal was called Second Nature. In 1990, we recorded a demo called "I Got It Goin' On," with producer and rapper Jermaine Dupri, who was then best known for working with Kris Kross and Silk Tymes Leather, and for being a dancer for the rap group Whodini. The idea was that we could use the demo to get signed, but it was never actually released. In the studio, Jermaine told me I should sing in a deep register all the time and make that my thing. I used to sing background vocals for Kris Kross's demos when Jermaine was trying to get them a record deal, and I felt like he had a good sense of my skill. I took his advice to heart. So every day Second Nature practiced and sang and danced in Crystal's house, hoping it would lead us to fame.

During all this, I was still working at the salon and learning how to do hair from a guy named Maurice Beaman and a woman named Marie Davis. I'd known Marie since I was 14 years old. I met her in a Kroger grocery store. She approached me and asked me to model for her salon.

"Let me ask my mom," I said.

Marie told my mama that I had a beautiful face. "There's something special about her," Marie said. So my mama let me start modeling for the salon in my teens. I won all the competitions they entered me in and it was only natural that Marie would eventually have me start learning to do hair myself.

She always said, "T, you gonna be a star."

"Girl, that's right!" I replied. "You can see it? 'Cause I be telling everybody and they don't believe me."

"Yes," she said, smiling. "You're a star."

Marie told me about a woman named Pebbles who had just moved to Atlanta with her husband L. A. Reid, a well-known record producer and the cofounder of LaFace Records with Kenny "Babyface" Edmonds. One day, standing in the beauty salon, Marie offered up some new information.

"You know," she said, "Pebbles is looking for a group."

"Well, go tell her I'm the bomb," I said recklessly. "Tell her she needs to holler at me."

That night my phone rang.

"Hello?" I answered.

"Is this Tionne?" It was Pebbles. I couldn't believe it. I was just talking junk, never thinking she'd actually call.

"Yes," I said. I stood in my room, holding the phone to my ear, shocked.

"Marie told me I should call you," Pebbles said. "I want to meet you."

She didn't waste any time. The next night Pebbles took me, Lisa, and Crystal to dinner at an Italian restaurant—nothing super ritzy—and got to know us. I thought Pebbles was so pretty. Everything she had was nice—thick, pretty hair, beautiful clothes, a fancy car. She even had a Chanel bag. She seemed nice, too. She was the sort of person who made you admire all the things she had—at least at first.

When my friends found out I was going to audition for Pebbles, they had a lot to say. Pebbles had a hot song out called "Mercedes Boy," which I loved at the time.

"You have to go in there and wear high heels and look like her," one said.

"She's all dolled up and she's high-class," another told me. "She's sa'diddy."

This was the term everybody used in Atlanta around that time to describe someone like Pebbles. If someone was super glamorous and wealthy, you'd call them "sa'diddy."

But I wasn't about to change who I was just to impress someone. "No," I told them. "She's gonna respect me for being myself. I'm gonna rock my stuff and show her who I am."

On the third night after Pebbles called me at home, we auditioned for her. I wore baggy jeans and a giant T-shirt. No high heels. Lisa and I went all in. Crystal, though, barely moved or sang. She just kind of stood there. But Pebbles told us she wanted us to be her new girl group anyway, despite Crystal's lazy effort. She even had a name for us: TLC. Each letter stood for the first initial of each of our names, which we thought was clever and fun.

The strangest part about the story of TLC, for me, is that I felt like I knew it was going to happen. I'd dreamed my entire life of performing on a stage in front of thousands of screaming fans, and I felt like that was inevitable for me. Two weeks before Pebbles called me, I felt it stronger than I ever had. I came home one day and told my mama, "I feel it. It's about to happen."

"What's about to happen?" she asked.

"I'm 'bout to blow up," I replied. I was so sure. "I'm 'bout to be on TV soon. I can tell."

My mama just smiled and said, "Okay." That was always her response when I said something like that. She said that as long as I kept my morals, integrity, and character intact, she'd support anything I did. She'd tell me, "Always be the best at whatever you do."

But I knew what was coming, whether she believed my premonition or not. Soon after I told her it was about to happen, Pebbles hollered at me and TLC came into the world. It felt like fate was guiding me.

As soon as Pebbles took control, it became clear that she wasn't a fan of Crystal. And, to be fair, Crystal wasn't a good fit. She still just stood there while we rehearsed, barely moving, not dancing at all. She once told Lisa and me, "I don't like to sing in front of people." But we were so young—I was 19 at the time—and we didn't exactly know how to control our own circumstances. But you have to have standards for quality—otherwise what are you even doing?

One day, before she officially signed us, Pebbles sat Lisa and me down in her office.

"Crystal's lacking," she said. "One can mess it up for the whole group."

We didn't know what to say, but we knew what she meant. She never said the words directly or told us we had to fire Crystal. But she hinted strongly.

We wanted Pebbles to be the one to send Crystal packing since it was her idea, not ours. But apparently it was our responsibility. Pebbles pulled us aside again, soon after the first conversation, and was more stern about it this time.

"If you don't get rid of Crystal, all of you are out," she said. No hints this time. We had to step up.

Lisa and I showed up at Crystal's house shortly after that. On the porch, just before we knocked on the door, I grabbed Lisa's arm. "Do you fight?" I asked. "Because we're about to throw her out of her own group, and if she gets rowdy, we're going to have to fight." Lisa nodded.

After Crystal let us in, we sat across from her at the booth in her kitchen. Lisa delivered the blow.

"Girl," Lisa told Crystal, "we got some good news and some bad news. The good news is that Pebbles wants to sign us. But the bad news is, girl, that we don't want you in the group no more."

I busted out laughing. I couldn't believe she said it like that. Crystal didn't try to fight us, though. She took the news really well and asked us to leave, wishing us luck on our way out. It was one of the hardest things I've ever had to do. But Pebbles's words lingered in my mind: "One can mess it up for the whole group."

As we walked out of the house and onto the front porch, we both felt a wave of relief. I felt bad for her, but we had to do what was right for us. It was our first important lesson: You have to put yourself first, be your own priority, and leave behind those who can't quite cut it. It's not selfish if it's the right thing to do for your career and you're not dogging someone out in the process. You have only one shot, and you have to take it. You just have to try not to burn any bridges along the way. Pebbles bought Ian out of his management position in February of 1991, officially signed us to Pebbitone Management, and it all began.

We held auditions to find a new member. We needed

someone who was a certain height, a certain look, and was able to sing and dance. It seemed impossible. But L.A. and Baby Face's record label, LaFace Records, had a new group called Damian Dame. This girl named Rozonda was dancing for them, and L.A. suggested her to Pebbles. In April of 1991, Pebbles brought her in, and the night we met her, we all rehearsed a song and a dance routine in the Pebbitone office. We christened her Chilli, our new "C."

The three of us went to the massive, gated house in Atlanta's Country Club of the South, where Pebbles and LA lived, to audition for L.A. and Dallas Austin, whom I knew from Jelly Bean's, and one of their producers, Kayo. The house was enormous. Usher actually ended up buying it years later. Driving through the neighborhood, I didn't find it hard to imagine myself in one of these giant mansions. I kept thinking, "I can't wait to live like this one day."

We walked into the house through the double doors. Inside everything was done up in natural tones. A balcony hovered high above us, leading onto the second floor. There was a real pretty dining room and this ornate fabric gathered together above the table at the chandelier. I thought, "Wow. This is how ballers do. I can't wait to get one of these one day." It wasn't that I wanted Pebbles and L.A.'s house or their actual stuff—I wanted my own version of it. I wanted to be the sort of person who would have a fancy dining room with a chandelier. It gave me the push to really work hard. I figured if I could prove myself and become a famous musician, then I could be a baller, too.

Each of us had prepared a song for the audition. Chilli sang "Hold On" by En Vogue, Lisa offered up an original rap, and I reprised "Wanna Get with U" by Guy. It was the perfect song for me—it showed off that low tone in my voice. All together, the three of us brought varied skills to the table. You could hear our different voices and tones in the audition, and you could tell how they might all work together. It felt like a success. It was intimidating, sure, but I had to seem confident. When we finished, L.A. simply said, "I like them."

So Chilli was in, and we officially signed as TLC with LaFace that summer. One of the first things Pebbles did was send me into a rehearsal space to figure out who I was going to be onstage. I selected the name T-Boz as my stage name. It started just as Boz, but I liked the idea that T-Boz was short for "Tionne is boss." It felt like it fit me. Pebbles put me in that rehearsal hall for 8 hours every day for 5 days straight, leaving me alone with myself and giving me food, water, and Gatorade.

"Go in there and figure out who T-Boz is," she said.

So I stood in that room, in front of the mirrors, and I figured it out. I had to find out how I was going to move, how I was going to look, and what my dances would be. Doing that made me raw. And throughout the years I just perfected it. I've always had my own signature moves. I grab my crotch when I dance. I roll my neck—people would talk about the T-Boz neck roll. Being in the rehearsal space on my own really made me identify who I was as an artist. I don't recall the other girls being sent in to do the same—maybe Pebbles was putting more pressure on me because I was leading the songs. But either way, after that, I was ready to go.

Almost immediately after we signed with LaFace, TLC went into the studio to make our first album with these mega-huge producers—Jermaine Dupri, Dallas Austin, Daryl Simmons, Kenny "Babyface" Edmonds. We recorded a lot of the tracks with Dallas at Doppler Studios in Atlanta. We were so hyped to be making our first album.

But despite all the excitement and the seemingly fairy tale direction my life was headed in, I was constantly sick from my disease. I got sick every 3 months, at least. If I overdid it at Jelly Bean's or if it was too cold outside that night, I'd be in pain that night or the next morning. If I rehearsed too hard, my limbs would ache. I always pushed through it, ignoring the pain and forcing myself to be the performer I wanted to be despite my illness—or, at least, until my body just collapsed and couldn't take it anymore. I refused to believe that anything could stop me from becoming T-Boz.

But soon after we went into the studio, I had a major flare-up of my disease. I was in pain all over my body and couldn't leave my bed. Lisa and Chilli called me from the studio after they'd laid down the tracks for our first single, "Ain't 2 Proud 2 Beg," which Lisa wrote with Dallas.

"T," Lisa said over the phone, "listen to this shit. It's so dope."

They played the song for me through the phone lines. I was so excited about it—it was a great song—but it was hard being trapped in bed by this disease. I was so sick. I couldn't be there in the studio and there was nothing I could do but wait to get better.

The pain eventually went away after I was released from the hospital yet again and I took care of myself like my mama and I always did. I got to go back into the studio, and the excitement returned. I wasn't a patient anymore. I was T-Boz, and I was making my first album.

We were so excited and we used to get really wild

between sessions, unable to control our energy. That turned into the most intense food fights you've ever seen—and I mean that literally. We threw food everywhere, at each other and at Dallas.

One night while in the studio, we got so out of control that the food fight took over the entire building. We wanted revenge on Dallas for the last fight, which we'd lost badly. Lisa had a plan: Mix flour and water together in a bowl and dump it on his head when he wasn't expecting it. But Lisa mixed it up too thick, and instead of running all over his head, the dough just stuck in the bowl on top of his head. He wasn't going to let us get away with that. Every time we grabbed some food and tried to hurl it at him, he'd grab our hands and mash the food in our faces with our own hands. We chased Dallas through the studio, from the recording control room into the halls, hurling water and food everywhere. Water pooled all over the floor. Ketchup, smashed sandwiches, and all kinds of food smeared the walls. To make matters worse, we poured water down the hallway so we could slide down it, like a really ghetto waterslide.

The people who ran Doppler Studios freaked out. They called Pebbles and LaFace. "You're going to have to pay for this damage," they told us. "Clean it up."

Eventually we calmed down, cleaned up the studio, and washed the walls. Dallas even had to clean the carpets with a rented shampoo machine. It took hours before we could go home. We were so bad. Looking back, I'm so embarrassed. My mama definitely taught me better than that.

But it was all in good fun. We were too young to really realize that time in a studio costs a lot of money and we were wasting it on food fights. I didn't yet understand the value of time in the music industry. Work and play should be kept separate, even if you have fun getting the job done.

We had a real goal with the music. We didn't necessarily aim for a specific genre. What made us unique was the combination of sounds, joining our three very different musical sensibilities. I was funk, Lisa was hip-hop, and Chilli was R&B, and it all surprisingly happened to cross over into pop. Together we made something that felt both familiar and new. Our chemistry together was amazing, the sort of thing that couldn't be bought or manufactured. Our songs were immediate, pounding with hooks, and broke new ground.

We were always passionate about having strong lyrical content, even from the start. The thing that made us so special was that we talked about relatable issues in our music and we did it in a fun way. We wanted to introduce the lyrics in a really danceable way. Every hook had a dance, so you'd always remember it—and the message, too.

Our first album, *Ooooooohhh . . . On the TLC Tip*, dropped on February 25, 1992, on LaFace/Arista Records. The title of the album came from the last line of the first single, "Ain't 2 Proud 2 Beg." I'll never forget the day it came out. We were in the parking lot at Taco Bell and "Ain't 2 Proud 2 Beg" came on the car radio. We were in Chilli's Volkswagen, which had a hole in the floor on the passenger's side. Stuff was always falling out of the hole while she was driving. We were pulled over at the Taco Bell, and our own voices blared out of the car speakers. All three of us leapt out of the car and started high-fiving and dancing in that parking lot. We didn't care who was looking.

"Ahh, shit!" Lisa said. "We 'bout to blow up!"

"We on the radio!" I screamed.

We were all over that parking lot, shrieking and jumping up and down. I couldn't believe that my voice was actually coming out of the car speakers. This was it. This was our moment. It was the beginning and I could feel it.

After it dropped, our album started climbing the charts. "Ain't 2 Proud 2 Beg," which first came out in November the year before, made it to No. 6 on the *Billboard* Hot 100 and "Baby-Baby-Baby," the album's second single, hit No. 2. The album itself made it to No. 3 on the *Billboard* R&B Albums chart, which was insane to us. Fame was coming. We'd never even played a real show.

But I remember the first real time TLC went onstage like it was yesterday. It was June 6, 1992. We were invited to open for MC Hammer on his tour, which was a big deal. Most artists start off with some club shows in smaller rooms—and we did do some college auditorium dates—but we catapulted right into arenas. Our first show on the tour was in Dallas at the Reunion Arena. Boyz II Men and Jodeci were also opening for Hammer. The tour had been going on since April, and when we arrived to join, it felt like we were really hitting the big time.

By the time we got to Las Vegas, a few weeks later, the whole world was buzzing about us. That night, June 26, was the first time we could feel the world responding to us. Apparently, everyone wanted to see these new TLC girls. Before the show started, I stood backstage, pacing around with Lisa and Chilli. It was unlike anything we'd ever seen: dressing rooms, catering, free snacks, people everywhere. Atlanta seemed really far away.

We were like racehorses, reeling toward the gates, ready

to run. Anxiety coursed through me, confused, in moments, with excitement. I felt urgently like I had to pee, but couldn't go. I hovered over the dressing room toilet uselessly. It's something that still happens to me every time I play a TV show—the nerves shoot through your body and give you all these mixed signals. I didn't think about how young I was or how inexperienced. I was just thinking, "This is it."

When I came back out, Jessica, our assistant, leaned over and reminded me to breathe. I tried to slow the air as it surged through my lungs, but it was impossible. This was our big moment. My heart pounded through my whole body. Thump thump thump.

We edged over to the side of the stage, getting ready to run out, and I could hear the crowd chanting. "TLC! TLC! TLC!" echoed through the venue, cried out by almost 20,000 people.

I grabbed Lisa's arm and gasped, "They're saying our name!"

"I know," she said excitedly. Her eyes were huge. I could tell she felt the same fear and excitement that I did. We'd never heard anyone shouting our own name back to us. It was crazy.

The chants got louder, rising through the room. All these people wanted to see us, three teenage girls from Atlanta. They knew our name. They loved us, already. I was already out of breath before we even got onstage.

And then we stepped out onto the expanse of the Las Vegas arena's stage, microphones in hand, and began to sing.

Later, I realized that show mirrored a dream I had had repeatedly as a kid. When I was 7 years old, growing up in Des Moines, I started having the most vivid dream. There was a stage and I was on the left side, wearing baggy pants and a baggy shirt. Below me, people screamed. I could hear nothing but their voices. In the dream, I had no face, like I was only seeing myself from the neck down, and I would run from the left side of the stage over to the right and gesture outward into the sea of people. It was always exactly the same. I had it constantly, for years and years.

It didn't mean anything at the time—it was just a dream I kept having. I didn't know it was offering me a real glimpse of my future, baggy clothes, left side of the stage, everything. I used to wake up and tell my mama, "People are going to know my name. They're going to know my face. I'm going to be on billboards and magazines across the world." She would just say, "Okay, sweetie." She heard me say it so many times. But I knew it was true.

I remember one time during high school a teacher asked us, "Where do you see yourself 10 years from now?" I blurted out, "On TV." Everyone laughed. I cried when I got home.

"Tionne," my mom said, "other people don't always believe in your dreams the same way you do. Sometimes you have to keep them to yourself and believe on your own." And I always did.

Onstage in Vegas, only a few weeks into our first-ever tour, with the crowd surging and chanting in front of us, everything was perfectly clear. You always hear people say, "My dream came true." It's a cliché, I know, but that's how it was for me. That night, I knew my dream had come true. TLC was going to make me a star.

CHAPTER 4

Running through the Halls

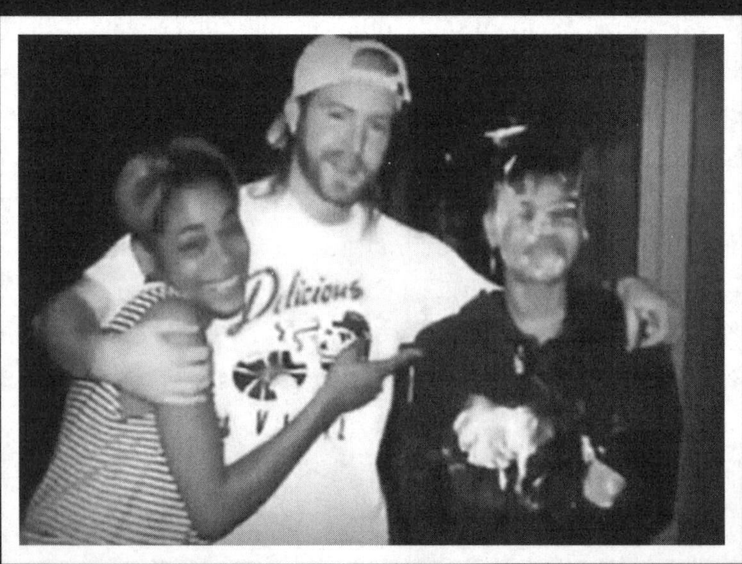

It's an amazing feeling to leave home and adventure out into the world with your band. I was happy to be there, but I didn't necessarily realize until I was older what an opportunity it is to get to see the world and all the awesome things it has to offer. When I was young, it was just about being in the moment. That was my attitude during the Hammer tour, which we had joined in Dallas in early June.

Boyz II Men and Jodeci were the other bands on the tour, and Dalvin DeGrate, known as Mr. Dalvin, was one of Jodeci's four members. I didn't notice him at first, not until he decided he wanted to talk to me. All of the dancers on tour loved him, and so did the groupies. Everyone used to whisper that the dancers were sleeping with the members of Jodeci, so I was wary of Dalvin. It wasn't until the end of the tour that we became friends—and then I started noticing how cute and fashionable he was. He had a good sense of humor, which is important to me. But as the tour kicked off, he was barely in my periphery. Plus, most of the guys who talked to us didn't care which member they got as long as it was one of us. That wasn't super comforting. So, instead, I focused my energy on TLC.

It was exciting to be so far away from home and from our former lives. No more hair salons. And none of us had traveled like this before. We quickly got used to the pace of touring, every day in a new town and everything constantly moving. Lisa, Chilli, and I went wild. We had been let loose into the world and we refused to be controlled. That meant, of course, that Pebbles didn't trust us when she wasn't there. She wanted to wrangle us at all times. She sent a woman named Joshlyn out on tour with us as our handler—which basically meant she was there to babysit us.

If we swore or misbehaved, Joshlyn would tell on us to Pebbles. Our pay for the week—already questionably low—would then get docked. You're kidding yourself if you think that stopped us from acting up, though. We still did whatever we wanted. We were three young adults on the road and wanted to take advantage of every opportunity to explore. But we were always being reminded that Pebbles was controlling our career.

Pebbles had this way of always making us feel like we weren't ever doing good enough. Maybe in her mind she was trying to make us better by always urging us to strive for something bigger. During the Hammer tour, we hit three million copies sold on our album. Our reaction? "That's the bomb!" Pebbles said, "Well, other people hit four million." Then we hit four million ourselves.

When we were happy with our success, Pebbles would always say something like that. "Well," she'd claim, "other people sold 10 million." Once we eventually hit 10 million, she said, "People like Whitney Houston have sold more than that with *The Bodyguard* soundtrack." I don't really know what her strategy was. Maybe she wanted us to have something to chase. She always made us feel like a kid who wants her parents' approval, but is never good enough. But honestly, it would push me to want to do better! And she would always tell me how fly she thought I was, which was comforting.

When the Hammer tour stopped in LA, we stayed at Le Montrose Suite Hotel near the Sunset Strip. We got tired of Joshlyn always trying to regulate us, so we hauled an ice bucket full of cold water up to her room. We banged our fists against the door, and when she opened it, her hair freshly permed, we hurled the water all over her head. It totally ruined her hair. We ran away, laughing.

We filled the ice bucket again and pounded on the door of a hotel guest who'd been playing guitar loudly in his room. You could hear it through the walls, and it was so bad.

"Room service," we shouted. When he opened his door, we doused him with the ice water, yelling, "Stop playing your fucking guitar!"

We took off down the halls convinced no one would ever catch us. Little did Chilli and I know Lisa snuck back and drew a left-eye symbol with an arrow on top of it using the sand from an ashtray in the hallway outside his room, marking her territory. Who does that? It was so funny, like a robber leaving a bank with a money trail scattered behind him leading right up to his front door. She was basically saying, "Hello! It was me!"

The next morning security kicked us out of the hotel. "This isn't appropriate behavior," they told us. We weren't that sorry, but we were allowed to come back only if we feigned an apology and promised to act better.

Hotel hallways were the place where we got into it. And we were in hotels an awful lot. Chilli and Lisa used to pull their butts out and run through the hallways to see if anyone would catch them. Butt cheeks out, flapping. Somehow they never got caught. But I didn't ever want to do it.

"You make me sick," Lisa said one night. "You won't never have fun with us. Pull your pants down!"

"You don't ever do it," Chilli agreed, jumping in.

"Shut up," I retorted. But I'd had enough of them nagging me. "Okay," I agreed. "I'll do it."

I yanked my pants down and started tearing down the hall, shrieking. I was running lopsided, trying to maneuver with my pant legs around my knees. I was freaked out someone in the hotel was gonna see me. A door opened. I turned around. It was our road manager, Woody, standing there, looking at my butt cheeks. I screamed and pulled my pants up. Lisa and Chilli were laughing so hard they could barely stand.

"See," I said to Lisa and Chilli. "This is why I don't do this."

But Lisa didn't stop. Another night she was skidding through the halls, pants down, and there was a turn in the corridor. Too late. Lisa didn't veer in time and she smashed directly into a giant mirror. It came tumbling off the wall and shattered all over her, like something out of a cartoon.

"Lisa," I said, "you're so clumsy." She was lying on the floor, glass everywhere, butt cheeks still drooping out of her pants. She ended up having to go to the hospital to get the mirror shards yanked out of her hand and a cut on her pinkie fixed. I sat with her in the room while a nurse came in to give her a shot and pull out the glass. When the nurse stuck the needle in Lisa's hand, blood shot everywhere and splattered all over the lady's face. Lisa and I laughed so hard. The nurse glared at us. If looks could kill, hers would have.

"Bitch, I ain't got AIDS," Lisa assured her. "You ain't gotta worry."

I was having a blast with Lisa and Chilli, and Dalvin was at the back of my mind. I knew he was cute and that girls liked him. It took weeks of touring before Dalvin and I started talking. He finally worked up the courage to approach me on the last week of tour, and we clicked right away. So by the end of the Hammer tour, he and I were dating. A lot has been written about me and Dalvin and our relationship. We used to have fun, but we argued a lot, too. We were really young—I was only 20—and we were both caught up in the throes of fame. He was popular, and he had girls coming at him every night. They'd just throw themselves at him. It's hard having a relationship when you're a celebrity in the public eye—and when you date a celebrity—that's one thing I'll say for sure. It feels like everybody's out to get you. But we liked each other, and he was important to me during this time, no matter the drama.

TLC had a lot of fun on that first tour, and it was exciting to be out on the road and to have this new boyfriend, but it was also incredibly difficult for me. I was sick off and on, and no one really knew how to help me. TLC was scheduled to perform at an awards show—I can't even remember which one because they've all blurred together—at one point during the tour, and I was super sick. One of Pebbles's staff members later told me that Pebbles didn't want to let me off the hook. "I don't care if she has to go out there and perform in a wheelchair, she's going onstage," Pebbles apparently said. I never found out if that was true, but it definitely didn't make me feel like she had my back.

I wasn't thinking a lot about my illness, though, mostly because I still didn't know how to manage it. I also didn't want to face the reality that I had the disease to begin with. My dreams were coming true, so sickness was the last thing on my mind. My mama had always told me that I could do whatever I set my mind to, and that's what I was trying to do. I never thought, "I'm sick, can I still do this?" I just assumed I could. I wasn't necessarily keeping my illness a secret, but my mentality was that my business was my business. I also didn't want anyone to pity me for something they'd never been through and that they didn't understand.

Unfortunately my body had other plans. Before one of our shows, I miscalculated my pain medicine and took too many pills. They had to do my makeup as I lay on the floor. I got dressed on the floor. I was carried to the edge of the stage for our performance, and our security stood around the stage to catch me in case I fell. After the show, I passed out and just lay there. People actually had to step over me. I felt done. I was so nauseated and messed up. My cousin Tae Tae, who danced for TLC, called my mom on the pay phone from the venue.

"You need to get here," she said. "She's not doing good." I ended up in the hospital after that show. My mom was there the next day.

Lisa and Chilli didn't know much about my illness. I fell ill and became weak and struggled to breathe and felt pain in my joints, but they didn't really get the severity of it. I didn't explain it, either. Dalvin didn't understand, either.

Everything came to a head after our show in Denver. I didn't know at the time that high elevation causes my disease to flare up. The lack of oxygen in the air thins my blood and I get really sick. As our tour bus pulled away from our show in Denver, I lay in my bunk and it felt like invisible knives were stabbing into me. I curled into a ball, clutching myself, hoping it would pass. I was in tears from the pain. When we arrived in Omaha, after a long, bumpy drive, they put me directly onto a stretcher and rolled me into the hospital.

My mama showed up immediately. She flew in and stayed by my side. It became clear to everyone that I was actually sick. This wasn't the flu or fatigue. I had a serious illness, and it was threatening my career. The doctor said I wasn't strong enough to continue on tour. TLC had to drop off and miss 2 weeks' worth of shows. I felt like there was a lot of weight on my shoulders because we were responsible for paying the crew and keeping all these people employed, and we were making no money during the downtime. Some people were furious that I was going to make us lose money. I'm sure they wanted me to keep going, but I couldn't. Lisa was concerned and supported me, so that was comforting and at least someone had my back!

That particular hospital experience in Omaha was really strange. A student got through security by posing as a doctor. He tried to check my pulse on my groin and kept trying to get a peek at my private parts. The police department had to scare away all the freaks by taking shifts outside my room. After I was discharged, my mom came back to get something from the hospital room and found a male nurse lying on my bed, sniffing the sheets. "This is where she was laying," he said. It was really spooky.

My health wasn't my only concern at the time. We started losing trust in Pebbles as the Hammer tour went on. We were worried about our contracts. One day, backstage, Lisa called me into the hallway.

She had been talking to some people who work with Hammer and wanted me to join in on the conversation. "They said we gotta pay more attention to how we gettin' paid." I nodded. Hammer's people would know how the business worked. If they said we should look into our contracts, then we should.

Even Hammer himself gave us that advice.

We started asking questions. But Pebbles didn't want to give us any answers. Whenever we asked her when we'd see some money, she'd reply, "The label has to recoup all the expenses first."

We started noticing differences between our career and those of other artists. If Pebbles wasn't the one to orchestrate a deal for TLC, then it wouldn't happen. It felt like she shut us down every time an opportunity arose outside of her.

Pebbles had been controlling from the start. Before Chilli joined up, Lisa and I took a trip out to Cali. Crystal had been kicked out by then, and Pebbles flew us out to dance in her video for her song "Backyard." Pebbles heard that New Edition MC Breed, Hammer, and some other bands were staying at our hotel, so she moved us to another one where they were having a retirement home staycation. Not as fun. There was a woman who worked for Pebbles named Tarryn who was supposed to look after us while we were out there. Lisa and I had no money, and we had to call home collect from the pay phones near the hotel. One day we called and asked Pebbles for 5 bucks apiece to buy some food from the Ralphs grocery store across the street. Instead of giving us the money, she had Tarryn take us to the store that was only across the street and buy us each exactly $5 of food. Tarryn was one of the cheapest people I'd ever met. She had a special wallet with categories for all the coupons. It was so weird to have someone control a few bucks to buy food. She could have at least handed us the money. How much could we have really balled out with $5 per person?

At one point I thought Pebbles and I were cool—we had grown close—but she was way too commanding. She always wanted to have "rap sessions" with us where she'd make us tell her our innermost secrets and problems. I already had a mother—and a great one at that—so I didn't need another. I didn't need her to be my psychiatrist or my Captain Save-a-Ho. I never got her motives, either. Right after our first album came out, Pebbles told me I needed to go solo. One day I was in her kitchen and Aaliyah's video for "Back & Forth" came on the TV. "See, T," she said. "That should be you." I didn't know what to say. I thought, "Does she really mean this or is she just looking for another payday? Because TLC just came out with their first album and she thinks I should be solo?"

She was notoriously jealous, especially where L. A. was concerned. After we finished shooting our video for "Ain't 2 Proud 2 Beg," Babyface and L. A. dropped by to congratulate us. As usual, we were broke and hungry. L. A. pulled out three $20 bills and handed one to each of us. Pebbles stepped over, snatched the money out of our hands, and said, "My man doesn't give any other woman any money." We were dumbfounded. There was no weird intent behind it. He was just trying to reward us for our hard work.

When Lisa, Chilli, and I confronted Pebbles about our contracts, she acted all hurt that we didn't trust her. But it was our legal right as the artist to see what we'd signed. We wanted to understand what the contracts said and how that affected us.

She put a wounded look on her face. "I have loved you and nurtured you like you were my own kids." And I was thinking what does that have to do with seeing our contracts.

Pebbles tried to keep the peace with us, especially after our album went platinum. She bought us each a car as a gift. It didn't really occur to us to ask where the money came from. But still, we kept realizing that other artists were seeing more of their profits than we were. Something definitely was amiss.

The three us went to see our lawyer and asked to see the contracts. We asked why we weren't making any money. He explained that Pebbles, Pebbitone, LaFace, and Arista were all getting a cut. And then we had management, legal, and accounting fees split three ways, as well as taxes.

It felt horrible. We had a platinum album. We were selling out shows, fans were mobbing us, and we had nothing to show for it. We suddenly realized that we'd paid for our own new cars, which we'd thought were gifts. Enough was enough. We were young, but we had to do better than this. The word *fair* has a different definition in our industry, especially if you've signed along the dotted line of a contract. No one cares what's morally right—morality goes right out the window. It's just about what you've signed and nothing else.

We met with L. A. and told him we didn't want to work with Pebbles anymore. He knew there'd been some drama going on between us for a while. He looked at us for a minute. "Well," he said, "you know she owns your name."

"Okay," we replied. "We'll buy it from her." We weren't going to give up our name.

"We want out," Lisa said, underscoring how important this was to us. He just nodded. We were going to do what we were going to do.

We ended up having to pay Pebbles $3 million for our name, $1 million for each letter. Even when we did make some money, it always seemed to have to go back to someone involved in the business, and this was another example of that. But it was worth it because it bought us some freedom. We couldn't completely rid ourselves of her since we were signed with Pebbitone through the record label. But Pebbles was no longer our manager after that.

It was the right thing for TLC to leave her, but everything Pebbles did wasn't awful. If it wasn't for her, I wouldn't have gotten my shot at stardom. I'll always be the first to admit that. She helped me identify who I was as an artist and as T-Boz. Even though I've lost a lot of respect for her over the years, I'd never erase her from my past. She's part of TLC's history. She made a difference in my life and in our band no matter our personal disagreements.

After we fired Pebbles, Hiriam Hicks became our new manager. We started to pay more attention. You have to notice things about everyone who joins your organization. If something is amiss, you need to move on again. We did that several times over the course of our career, but at that time Hiriam helped to push TLC forward.

With a new sense of freedom, TLC joined Bobby Brown on his tour, which kicked off in Charleston, West Virginia, in December of 1992. It was us, Shabba Ranks, and Mary J. Blige opening up for him. By that point we had more experience. We knew how touring worked and our shows had gotten tighter. I was still worried about getting sick, but I just kept hoping my body wouldn't fail me. I had to do this and I wanted it, so any discomfort was worth it. Sometimes I think about what I put myself through to do this. Another time, when we were on the Hammer tour, I didn't want to ruin the tour again by having to stop so I rode on the plane on a flight to Alaska for 22 hours during a sickle cell crisis. It was so painful that I remember hiding under my cover, pretending to be asleep and crying. I didn't make that show but at least we stayed on the tour.

Bobby had four dancers in his act. One of them—who we can call Alexis (not her real name)—had dated Dalvin, who was still my boyfriend, before me. She was a ho. She didn't like me and always started issues with me, which made me not like her, either. She and the other dancers in that crew had it out for TLC. But it was Alexis who especially didn't like us, and since she and some of the other girls were screwing the talent, they felt like they could do whatever they wanted—even antagonize us. Let's be clear, that's not typical hired-dancer protocol. Usually, if you mess with the artist, you get fired.

We didn't take any mess, not from dancers, not from hos, not from the label—not from anyone. We weren't necessarily cocky, but we were very confident. By the time we were on Bobby's tour, we were, like, "Yup, we're here. We're the jam." We had this slogan we used to shout onstage: "Look who runnin' thangs." We even had jackets that said it. We had our Wench Mob, which were our dancers, and our slogan and we thought we were doing it big.

There was a break in the tour dates for the American Music Awards, which took place on January 25, 1993. It was our first time at a serious awards show, and we were beyond excited. Getting dressed was a serious deal. We had to look fly and to make an impression. The other artists on the tour, Bobby and Mary J. Blige, were also nominated. We were up for Favorite Rap/Hip-Hop Artist and Favorite Rap/Hip-Hop New Artist. We lost Favorite Rap/Hip-Hop New Artist to Kris Kross, which didn't bother us much, but in the other category, we lost to Sir Mix-a-Lot, who had just come out with the song "Put 'Em on the Glass."

We did not handle that loss well. When they announced Sir Mix-a-Lot as the winner, we looked at each other, like, "What the fuck?" I mean, we lost at the AMAs to "Put 'Em on the Glass." Not even to "Baby Got Back." We were pissed. We desperately needed to blow off some steam.

When we got to the after-party, Lisa handed me a White Russian and one of those Dr Pepper shots that's lit on fire.

"Here," she said. "We need this."

I don't drink and alcohol doesn't mix well with my sickle cell disease. I also don't like the taste of alcohol. I had no idea what I was drinking or how much to drink or what it was gonna do to me. But I was on edge from the awards show, and I wanted to see what would happen. I drank both. I got tore up, fast.

Finally, Lisa hauled me away from the bar and out of the party. Everything looked blurry. I felt strange and my head was spinning. Lisa led me out the door of the party. As we exited, one of Bobby's dancers slammed into Lisa's shoulder.

"What the fuck?" Lisa said, turning around to face her.

The dancer balled up her fist and popped Lisa in her left eye. Alcohol is bad on so many levels. Everything felt like it was happening in slow motion. I didn't know what to do, and my reflexes were super slow. The dancer sauntered away.

"Lisa," I slurred, "she hit you in the eye!" Lisa clutched her face, furious. There was a line of red under her eye, like a blood vessel had burst. Our dancers ran up, ready to fight, but Bobby's crew of dancers had already run off.

When we got back to our hotel, I was sobbing hysterically. I was too drunk to really function, and I was so frustrated by the fact that I wanted to help Lisa. That heffa had hit her, and if you hit Lisa, it's like you've hit me. Our crew started mobilizing to go fight Bobby's crew, but I was too drunk to help. It was the only time in my life that I haven't been able to fight when I wanted to. Chilli; Marie, our hairstylist; Jessica, our assistant; and our dancers were ready to go. I tried to follow everyone out of the hotel. They sat me in a chair in the lobby, refusing to let me come.

"I'm sorry, Lisa," I muttered, tears streaming down my face. I felt so helpless.

Marlon Wayans came over to me where I was sitting in the lobby. He asked, "Are you drunk?" Yes, I was drunk. I nodded. What a way to meet someone for the first time! And me with an ugly cry going on.

Pebbles showed up and stopped the fight before it happened, even though she wasn't our manager anymore. That incident was how Lisa started drawing the line under her left eye. It started as a Band-Aid to cover up a burst blood vessel and later she turned it into a black mark. There's an origin story for everything, even if it's crazy.

Everything calmed down momentarily as we headed back on the road. The tour kicked off again in Albany, and there was over a month left of shows. But a few days later, Lisa showed up in our dressing room. She had a box in her hands, and she looked like she was on a mission.

"What's that?" I asked. Lisa slapped the box down on a table and opened it. She looked pleased with herself. Inside the box there was a brand-new .22 gun.

"I'm gonna shoot that bitch," she said. She meant the dancer who'd popped her in the eye.

"What?" I said, shocked. I fight, and I'll always throw down when warranted, but this seemed kinda extreme.

"Yep," Lisa confirmed, "I'm gonna shoot her."

Our management had to intervene. They took the gun away from Lisa, which she protested loudly.

"I'm not going to kill her," Lisa said. "I was just gonna shoot her in the knee or the toe or something."

"No," everyone said unanimously. "You can't shoot her at all." But we were only halfway through the tour, and something had to be done to keep the dancers away from us. So management divided the arenas in half every night from then

on. We had to stay on one side of the line, and the dancers had to stay on the other. It got really messy. Security would escort Bobby's dancers to and from the stage before and after his performances.

Our own dancers had started getting involved, too. They carried around these miniature bats. Once Tae Tae took her bat and smacked one of Bobby's dancers in the kneecap. Tae Tae wanted to give her a warning, like, "We'll fuck you up if you mess with TLC." And Tae fights like two men combined, so you don't want to mess with her.

Another day, Chilli ran breathlessly into our dressing room and announced, "Two of them just surrounded me. One was in the front and one was in the back." She grinned and added, "But I stood my ground. I ain't scared. I'll fight those bitches." And she would have, too.

We tried to tell Bobby that his girls were out of line, but he and his brother Tommy loved them. The three of us met with Bobby and Tommy and asked for his help.

"These hos are getting out of line," Lisa said.

"They're taking it too far," I added. Bobby said he would talk to them, but we got the sense that nothing was gonna change, since they were sleeping with those girls. We had to stick to our side of the arena, and those heffas had to stick to theirs.

That was one of the best tours I've ever been on, but it was also one of the most chaotic, dramatic, and messy. It was second only to the Hammer tour, which is still my favorite tour I've ever been on. And, despite the drama, I loved every minute of the Bobby Brown tour. Marie, the same Marie who'd started this all back in Atlanta, was along for the ride to do our hair, and some of my funniest stories involve her. We

started pranking each other on the road, always trying to one-up what the other person pulled. It started innocently, with a food fight. I honestly don't know why we were always flinging food around.

One night Belinda, our road manager, came into the dressing room with this piece of chocolate cake. "Nobody eat my chocolate cake," she told us. "I'm not playing. Catering has no more cake. Don't let anybody touch my cake. Don't." She wrote her name on the plate and left it on a table.

When I walked into our dressing room after coming off stage, Marie hurled something at me. It was a piece of food. I threw some back at her. We ended up throwing everything in there. There was food all over the dressing room, and I had food covering my face. Eventually, we ran out of stuff to throw. That's when I saw Belinda's cake.

"You better not," Marie warned. But I took that cake and chucked it at Marie's face. Chocolate smeared all over her. Belinda walked in the room and I immediately shouted, "Marie stole your cake."

"Marie!" Belinda said. She looked pissed. I kept a straight face, but Marie started laughing. "I didn't," Marie protested.

"Yes, you did, Marie," I accused. I was trying not to laugh.

"Belinda," Marie said, "she threw ya' cake." Belinda couldn't tell who was telling the truth. She was so mad. She stomped out. But I think she believed me.

Marie got me back soon after. Everyone knows how I am about my hair, especially her. You'll never see those big Michael Jackson fans on our stage blowing my hair around. I don't like my hair to blow or even to move. Right before I go onstage, I always take the comb from the hairstylist and make a few adjustments. My hair has to be 100 percent

perfectly shaped, especially my sideburns. So one night right before we about to walk onstage at an awards show to accept an award, Marie came over to me. She took both her hands and roughed up my hair. "Bye," she said. "Have a nice show."

That year TLC was asked to shoot some scenes for *House Party 3*, which came out in early 1994. We played a fictional band called Sex as a Weapon and it was so much fun. On the set, Marie went up to Chuckii Booker and told him I wanted to sleep with him. She told him in front of all his friends, so they all thought I was after him. I had no idea. Marie kept asking me to do this nasty gyrating dance, goading me to do it. I didn't notice it was right in front of Chuckii.

"Hey, T," she said, "do that dance for me." Here I was dancing all nasty, and he thought I was doing it for him. Marie let it go on until we left for the day. She told me after he was gone. That heffa. This went on for years. We pranked each other all the time. It kept things fun. It reminded us that we were still normal people who liked to have a good time and to laugh. We weren't exactly normal people in the eyes of the public by that point, so it was important to remind ourselves.

There's this thing that happens when you start learning you're becoming famous. You see people's reactions to you when you're not onstage, and you just know. One day, before a show on the tour, we went to a mall somewhere in the Midwest. We wanted to shop, but we started getting recognized. People formed a crowd and chased us. They formed a mob. It was so scary.

We started going places and people would rock the car and not let us drive away. That was when we realized we'd made it. We did a one-off tour date in Jamaica, and afterward fans mobbed the car. We were stuck there for almost an hour, not moving. They had to get all the kids off the car so we could leave. It's really weird when you experience it for yourself. At first you smile because you realize, "Oh we're famous." Then you realize someone could get very hurt. I've had fans rip strands of my hair out so they could have a piece of my infamous sideburns, and I've had my earrings snatched out of my ears. They wanted to keep something of mine, whatever it could be.

One night a fan fainted when I came onstage. It's weird to see people drop like flies when you step out in front of them. I was her favorite band member, so after the show, as she was lying on a stretcher, I went to say hello. I touched her leg and she started hyperventilating. She almost stopped breathing completely. It was insane. The paramedics had to send me away so they could work on her. I was so upset and became nearly hysterical myself because I'm just a person. To this day it makes me uncomfortable when people cry over me. But I know, to them, I'm more than I used to be.

Our most infamous fan encounter happened in April of 1993. We were booked to play a show at Six Flags Magic Mountain in Southern California. The show was supposed to take place 3 days after the verdict came in for the Rodney King federal civil rights trial. Tension in Los Angeles and around the country was high. Race was an issue, and everyone was worried about more riots. The show was us and Paperboy, and Magic Mountain couldn't handle the massive number of fans who wanted to come.

The concert tickets sold out almost immediately, and the fans, many of whom were already inside the amusement park, were not happy about it. They'd come to see us, and the park wasn't letting them. So they rioted. Hundreds of people tore the park up, breaking windows and looting the shops. Then they tore up the surrounding area in Santa Clarita. A nearby Wendy's had all of its windows broken, and people smashed in the salad bar and the cash registers. There was a lot of damage, and the cops started arresting people. They had to bring out the National Guard to escort us back to the hotel. They walked alongside our van with massive rifles as the driver steered us out.

Back in our hotel, which was around the corner from Magic Mountain, we didn't realize that the rioting had continued into the night and next morning until rocks started crashing through our hotel room windows. Lisa and I woke up to glass shattering. The fans didn't know we were the ones in the hotel—they just wanted to destroy anything they could find. We had to be escorted out of the hotel.

The next day, the news had a field day with the incident. We got blamed, even though it wasn't our fault that the promoter had oversold the concert. Magic Mountain spokeswoman Eileen Harrell told the *Los Angeles Times* that the crowd rioted because they were attracted by "that type of music," calling us a rap group. TLC isn't a rap group, as anyone who's a fan of us knows. She also said, "We won't be scheduling any more groups like that in here, ever." She made it a race thing, which was ignorant and unfortunate because our audience was totally mixed. We've always had fans from all races, including white, black, Hispanic, and Asian. We're universal, so it was gross the way they spun it.

The writer of the *Los Angeles Times* news article wrote, "The two groups that performed are regarded as milder than the hard-core 'gangsta' rap groups more commonly associated with violence at concert venues." If someone wrote that about an artist now, there would be an uproar.

But the flip side was, after that, we knew we were really popular. We'd become massively famous, and fans would cause a scene if they weren't allowed to see us. We didn't always know whether something should or shouldn't be happening. We just rolled with it. We were always excited to be involved and to be there, whatever it was. It felt like a big party all the time, even when things got scary or the fans mobbed us.

We got to go to the Grammys for the first time in February of 1993, right before the tour with Bobby Brown wrapped. "Ain't 2 Proud 2 Beg" was nominated for Best R&B Song. We didn't win, but it was worth it to get to be there. That was the night I met one of my favorites, Patti LaBelle. I grew up loving her because of my mom. She was at the RCA Records Grammys after-party, and I was so happy. We were hopping from party to party, taking full advantage of our nomination, and I saw her from across the room.

"Oh my God," I said to Patti, awed. "I love you. My mama loves you. I'm so excited to meet you." She gave me the biggest hug. The next time I saw her, she sang one of my lyrics back to me. It was everything. Patti LaBelle knew who I was, and she sang my song and sounded just like me. Even when you become famous yourself, the truth is that you can still get excited over other celebrities.

Our first album felt like a giant whirlwind that lasted nearly 2 years. I remember working constantly, barely taking any time off to come home. After the Bobby Brown tour wrapped, and after we finished all the extra shows they'd booked for us, it was finally time to go home to Atlanta. It was time to make our second record, and now the pressure was on.

CHAPTER 5

Crazy Sexy Cool

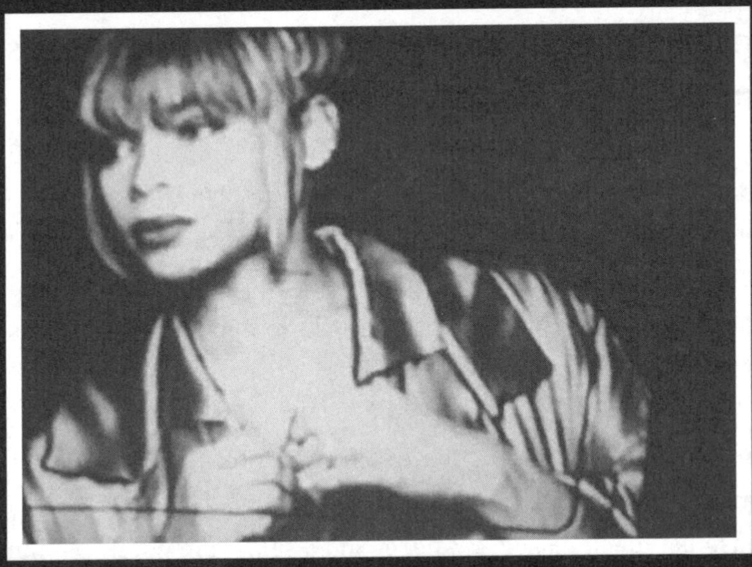

After we got off tour for *Ooooooohhh . . . On the TLC Tip*, we were living large. It was the first time the three of us had a break since the album exploded on the scene, and we were just young and famous enough to get into trouble and experience some things. As I was resting and getting my personal life back in order, Lisa moved herself into her boyfriend Andre Rison's massive house.

Andre played for the Atlanta Falcons, and they'd started dating just after our album had dropped. Their relationship was full of love and drama. By the summer of 1994, Lisa had already filed one assault charge against Andre, which he'd denied. None of it was going anywhere good. They had this weird love/hate thing going on, like, "I can talk about you, but no one else can."

On June 9, 1994, I got a call from Pebbles. Lisa had been arrested for burning Andre's house down. The night before Lisa had been pissed at Andre. She'd said, "I'm gonna get my girls and we gonna get dressed up and we gonna stay out later than him." But when Lisa came home, Andre and his boys were still out clubbing. And she was mad.

When she came home that night, Lisa saw stacks of brand-new sneakers in the house, with none for her. Lisa took all those Nikes into his bathroom, threw them in the bathtub, and lit them on fire. But here's the thing: This wasn't the only time she'd started a fire. The first time it had been a bunch of stuffed animals in the bathtub, and Andre had replaced the original bathtub with a Plexiglas one. So when she lit the sneakers, the whole thing was like "Whoosh!" and the entire house went up in flames.

Meanwhile, Lisa told me she had written a letter in red lipstick around the whole room, literally from the top of the wall to the floor. That was my girl—she always had the best ways of getting back at people. That letter burnt up with the rest of the house, so only Lisa knew what it said. She was one of the funniest people I ever met. When I got the call that she'd been arrested, I wasn't that surprised. I'd gotten these kinds of calls before: "Tionne, can you come get Lisa? She's running naked in the woods." I don't know what it was about Lisa, but she loved to get butt-naked when she was drunk. So I'd go haul her out of the woods and make her put a blanket or her clothes back on.

For some reason, Lisa always listened to me. Before I'd get there, she'd be yelling and swinging at people, but if I said, "Lisa, you butt-naked in the woods—come in the house," she'd just reply, "Okay," like a sweet, big-eyed baby girl. I loved her eyes. They always got me.

The morning of the fire, when I got the call, I asked, "Is she okay?" Yes, she was fine. She'd run out the house after setting the fire and fought with Andre in the driveway. She was bruised up, and some of her nails were coming off. She hadn't bashed in the car windows, even though she was blamed for it. Andre's friends were mad at Lisa for starting the fire, so they'd bashed in her car windows to get even. The news blamed everything on Lisa. Ultimately, though, a house is just a house. It's a horrible thing to lose, but with insurance and those football funds, Andre would bounce back. I hope he didn't lose anything sentimental.

"Well, where is she?" I asked. She was at a hotel. Me and Chilli went there to sit with her until the label and the lawyers could figure out what to do. She later turned herself in and was arrested. The news was everywhere, immediately. Andre did an interview with *People* 2 weeks after the fire and told them that Lisa had a drinking problem. This meant that TLC's name was all over the papers and in every news report. We were on CNN every day. But then O. J. Simpson drove his white Bronco away from the cops, and it finally took the shine off Lisa. I called my mama, "We ain't on TV no more because O.J. did something." But the damage had been done. No one wanted to work with TLC after Lisa burned the house down. They didn't want us wearing their clothes, nothing. In their eyes, if one of us did something wrong, then all of us had messed up.

Lisa was sentenced to 5 years of probation and court-ordered alcohol rehab. The judge also handed her a fine of $10,000 for first-degree arson. A week later she went into a diversion center to do her time. Lisa asked me not to come see her in the diversion center. I followed her wishes. She seemed to want to keep that part of her life separate. I remember her telling me later how mean the lady there was to her. She was forced to do disgusting things just because she was a celebrity, like clean the floor with a toothbrush. Lisa was stuck in there, but the world was waiting for a second TLC album. So while Lisa was in rehab, Chilli and I went back into the studio.

We'd started working on our second album at the end of 1993, but now we were behind schedule. We worked with Babyface, Dallas, and Jermaine again this time around. We weren't always in the studio together—especially since Lisa was AWOL—but we knew what we wanted from these new songs.

Once you succeed, you don't necessarily know how you did it. It was just something that happened organically. So after that, we had to step back and try to figure out what we did right the first time so we could do it again. We knew our hooks were good, and we knew it was important to keep talking about real issues in the songs. People liked us because we made unique-sounding tracks that actually had strong lyrical content and a dance to every hook and chorus. Now we needed to decide who we were going to be the second time around.

I can't tell you how many songs we tried until we found the vibe that we liked. I remember singing a song called "Leaving Las Vegas" that didn't make it. It just wasn't quite right. I went through a lot of tracks trying to find how we were going to sound. There's all kinds of unreleased demos of me singing stuff, figuring out the vibe. Ultimately, we found it on songs like "Creep" and "Waterfalls." "Creep" actually started out as a solo song for me, which was written about a situation between me and an ex-boyfriend, but became one of the central tracks on *CrazySexyCool.*

By then Dallas had bought his own studio in Atlanta,

DARP Studios, and we laid down most of the tracks there. Most of the time, it was me, Dallas, and Leslie Brathwaite in the studio. Leslie was our runner until one day the engineer didn't show up.

"Dallas," I said. "Leslie can do it." Leslie looked surprised. He just stared at me wide-eyed. But I knew he could do it. He had spent countless hours behind the soundboard after our sessions. That night he became my new engineer. He's since worked with Madonna and Michael Jackson, Jay Z, Beyoncé, Pharrell, and Mariah Carey as well as in movies like *Transformers*—you name it—and I helped induct him into the Full Sail University Hall of Fame, where he'd graduated alongside many greats. He's now my best friend, my daughter's god daddy, and one of the best engineers in the business.

I sang most of *CrazySexyCool* in the studio by myself with only Dallas and Leslie there. The interludes between the songs felt really important on this album. We had to get them right. They wanted us to record them with Sean "Puffy" Combs, so the label flew us to New York to record with him. I'd worked with Puffy before, but unfortunately we hadn't seen eye to eye. I'd recorded a song with him, and it had ended in a near fight.

"I'm gonna take this back to Dallas and do it with him instead," I'd told Puffy in the studio the first time around.

"Fuck that," he replied. "This was my idea." We got up in each other's faces. We looked like we were about to fight. Jessica calmed me down.

"Screw this," I said, and left. I flew back to Atlanta and went straight to Dallas.

"I'm doing this with you," I said. "Not Puffy. He didn't

understand how to work with me, and I didn't understand his methods, either."

L. A. had to step in and convince me that we could meet in the middle. I could record my part with Dallas, and then Puffy could come to Atlanta to produce the record with his own producer Chucky Thompson and Dallas. That's what we did, and it became a remake of "If I Was Your Girlfriend" by Prince. Afterward, Puffy and I made up. TLC went to New York to record our interludes with him, and we became known for those after *CrazySexyCool* dropped.

Lisa had to come out of rehab to record her vocals for most of the album. She showed up one day with her rap for "Waterfalls," lyrics she'd started writing after seeing a rainbow. Chilli and I loved it immediately. "Waterfalls" was my way of trying to tap into alternative music. My boys from childhood, Rico and Marqueze Etheridge and their crew, Organized Noise, came up with the song, and it was amazing. We got CeeLo Green to sing the background vocals with Debra Killings.

The most important part of the song was that it had a message. AIDS was a big epidemic at the time. It was something that needed to be talked about. Us speaking about AIDS directly in a song made people feel like we were standing up for them. It also talked about the illegal drug trade and how a mother lost her son because of it. When you first come out as a band, you just hope people like you. But when you come out again, you have to evolve. You have to be better. We had relatable topics and memorable dances to each hook on the first album, but to talk about real social issues without sounding like we were preaching also helped push us to the next level.

When *CrazySexyCool* dropped on November 15, 1994, we'd already unveiled one single, "Creep." It was tough getting the video right for that one. And music videos are notoriously difficult. They look good, but making them is a trial by fire. It took us three tries to get the video for "Creep" right. We kept going back to the drawing board because the ideas weren't what we needed to hit big again. It was never good enough. The video for Salt-N-Pepa's "Whatta Man" had dropped right around the same time as our album. It was directed by a guy named Matthew Rolston. We decided we needed to get him to direct the "Creep" video. We were used to running our own stuff, so it was an adjustment.

Matthew was really hands-on. He did the clothing, the choreography—everything. TLC wasn't used to that. We had an argument over the wardrobe, and there was some tension over the dance moves for the video. I created the routine for "Creep." The funny part is that I will sometimes make up routines to other people's music, and I made up "Creep" to Dr. Dre's *The Chronic* album. When we got to rehearsal so I could teach the other girls my routine for the video, we were locked out of the space. There was this choreographer in there talking about how he already had our routine. This particular choreographer ended up becoming really famous for working with Beyoncé, but his claim to fame at the time was "Hold On" by En Vogue. We were like, "What? We do our own routines." We weren't sure why he didn't realize that and had us wait outside in the lobby.

"Look," I said, when we got into the rehearsal space. "I don't know how other groups work, but I think we work kind of differently." We looked at his routine, but of course we thought mine was better. That's what we used, although as a compromise I took two of his moves and added them to mine. As we practiced, the choreographer kept stopping us to fix things. Lisa got so mad.

"Why don't you do what you get paid to do, motherfucker,"

she snapped. "Push play and stop on the tape deck. Push play and stop. That's your job, not to be over here messing with me." *Motherfucker* was her favorite word at the time. The staff from LaFace were there, drinking gin and juice, and they were done. They thought it was hilarious, but very stressful.

There was another argument over the clothes.

"TLC is different," Lisa said. "You see that motherfuckin' sweater over there? T-Boz will make that a hat." She was talking off the top of her head. But her point was there: We were known for dressing differently. We ended up deciding to wear silk pajamas. They were custom made. It felt like our thing, and Matthew agreed to the compromise. It was embarrassing, though, because Lisa kept calling him a motherfucker throughout the shoot. It ended up being a phenomenal video. It was how we came back on the scene because it showed the growth of TLC. That was a big deal. We came from these tomboys to being more like sexy women. Matthew put a flash of my boobie cake in the video, and men still talk about it to this day. It helped reveal our womanhood.

The "Creep" video did really well and helped move the needle, but we didn't know "Waterfalls" would be the key to the album. I knew from the start that it was a good song and that it needed strong visuals. A video can make a song come alive and pop, and that's the kind of song "Waterfalls" was. Everybody could relate because it's upbeat sounding with massive, attention-grabbing horns, but it's also relatable to a certain group of people with its subject matter. But how do you make that subject interesting to everybody? You've gotta make it a strong visual message. Big, million-dollar videos weren't being made by everyone back then—it wasn't a thing yet. But we knew the song needed a massive music video to go along with it.

Clive Davis, then the founder and president of Arista Records, didn't like "Waterfalls." He just didn't believe it was a good song, and he didn't want to let us make the video we imagined. So we made this poster board, which was a written letter begging L. A. to give us a chance to shoot the video, and marched into L. A.'s office. We knew we wouldn't disappoint him.

"You've gotta believe in us," I said.

"We want you to front us the money for the video since Arista won't give it to us," Lisa added.

"If you believe in us, we'll make you the best video ever," Chilli said. We all nodded.

"All right," L. A. said. "I'll take your word for it." And he gave us the money, $1 million. He did believe in us. Later, he had that poster board framed for his office. We asked for F. Gary Grey to direct the video. We met with him and explained our concept, and it was immediately clear that he was the right person to bring it to life.

We filmed the video for "Waterfalls" on June 8 and 9, 1995, at Universal Studios Hollywood in the same place *Jaws* was shot. It felt like a big deal because it was the first time we were allowed to do the whole concept for one of our music videos. It all came together in unison.

The "Waterfalls" video was also the first time our stylist Julie Mijares started dressing us. She stepped in after we ditched our last stylist at a store by sending her in to buy clothes and then driving off. Before that stylist, I used to dress us. I'd fly to New York and buy clothing and material and sometimes Lisa would airbrush them or her uncle would sew them. Until Julie, stylists wouldn't last with us. Julie had done "Rhythm Nation" for Janet Jackson, and she was perfect for our trend-setting style. She dressed us far ahead of the rest of the music industry. She put us in futuristic clothes way before that look was poppin'.

On the day of the shoot, we had to start hair and makeup at 4:00 a.m. so that filming could start at 6:00 a.m. That meant we had to be up by 3:00 a.m. So the night before the shoot, they gave each of us a sleeping pill to make sure we would go to bed.

"Have your ass in bed by 8," management told us. "Your call time is 3:00 a.m." We were so bad that they had to treat us like kids. They didn't trust us to get enough rest on our own. I went to sleep at 8:30 p.m. and woke up on time at 3:00 a.m. to go to the shoot. They did our hair and makeup in trailers near the set, and as we were waiting to get started, we realized we didn't have a dance routine for the video. We hadn't had the time to practice one.

I made up the "Waterfalls" dance in my trailer that morning. There was a dance in Atlanta called the Bankhead Bounce, which is what inspired it. I thought, "Let me make a variation of that and slow it down, add a little something extra, and make it our own thing." I created that routine in about 10 minutes. Lisa and Chilli liked it, and we practiced it as quickly as possible. No one ever realized that I basically pulled it out of my ass on the spot.

So much work went into making the video over those 2 days. We had to stand on a thin, clear bar they'd built in 80 tons of water, and you had to take a boat to get to it. I can't swim, so there were six scuba divers under the water surrounding us just in case. I couldn't move forward or backward—that's why you see my feet anchored in. I could move only my arms and my midsection. The water swayed as we stood on the bar, and it was terrifying. You obviously couldn't wear a life vest. We got up there, did our new dance routine, and just hoped those scuba divers could catch me if I fell.

That day, I also found an opportunity to pay Marie back for all her pranks. Guess who showed up to the set of "Waterfalls"? Our old friend Chuckii Booker. Seeing him reminded me that I owed Marie for the stunt she pulled during *House Party 3*. I found the sloppiest, dirtiest guy in the video crew. He looked homeless. His fingernails were filthy and his breath stunk. It was perfect.

"Do you have a girlfriend?" I asked him. He shook his head no.

"Great," I continued, "because my hairstylist, Marie, is really shy and she likes you a lot." I handed him a note I'd written as if I was Marie. It had her cell phone number and hotel room on it and said, "Will you spend time with me?" He was thrilled. He sidled up to her trailer like a dirty pimp and said, "Hey, I got your note."

"I didn't write a note," she said.

"Tionne said you would say that," he replied. He called her a bunch of times and kept calling her hotel room. I couldn't resist. Even though all those years had passed, I owed her and it was worth it.

When we finished shooting the video, all three of us cried. It was the culmination of so much effort and so much passion. "It's so good," we agreed when we saw the first cut. "We don't even have to be in it!" And it wasn't just us who thought so. "Waterfalls" spent 7 weeks at No. 1 on the *Billboard* Hot 100, and the video won four awards at the 1995 MTV Video Music Awards, including Video of the Year. We became the first black artists to ever receive the trophy for that award. The video made was only the second music video by an African American artist played on VH1, after Michael Jackson. We've played "Waterfalls" so many times since, on massive stages and on TV shows around the world. It's our most influential song to this day. And it means so much to me because we believed in ourselves and our vision enough to fight for it. We got to be a voice during the AIDS epidemic, and that feels so important even now.

By 1995, TLC became one of the biggest bands in the world. *CrazySexyCool* was the fifth best-selling album of the year in 1995. Truth be told, some of Lisa's antics helped get our name out there even more. If you didn't know TLC for "Waterfalls," then you knew us as the group with the girl who'd burned down that football player's house. We appeared on the cover of *Vibe* magazine wearing firefighter outfits. The headline read "TLC Fires It Up," and the tagline said "Burning Up the Charts, Burning Down the House." Other magazines jumped onboard. *Rolling Stone* used "Burn, Baby, Burn" as their headline, writing "The women of TLC stay cool under fire." Everyone knew who we were, and they cared equally about us and about the music. Lisa even thanked the Atlanta Fire Department in an acceptance speech for one of the many awards we won for the album.

The success of our album gave us a lot of opportunities to be in the spotlight. I was invited to be the mistress of ceremony at the Rhythm & Blues Foundation Pioneer Awards, an event that was meant to highlight the past and future of the music industry. TLC, apparently, represented the future, so they had me come. Everyone was there: Prince, Smokey Robinson, Barry White, Stevie Wonder. It was amazing. They selected Aretha Franklin to represent the past. She and I were meant to stand onstage side by side and present during the ceremony. But she didn't want her podium next to mine.

I didn't even know her, so it was weird for her to diss me.

"Move my podium to the other side," she told the people organizing the event. What? She was an icon and acting crazy.

At the time, I was petite with meat. That means I was tiny, but with a little booty. They gave me a size 2 dress, one of those sample showroom ones, and it was see-through with slits covering your good stuff. I never came out in TLC dressed girly, so this was a first for the public. I was known for baggy pants, not gowns. Everyone was used to me looking like a boy. Aretha came out first. When I followed, the audience gasped. You could hear them saying things like "She looks so pretty. I didn't know she had a shape!"

"What?" Aretha said into her microphone. "You think she looks good? I used to look like that, but, uh, way better."

Was she serious? Anger swelled through me. I could feel my mama out there in the audience, praying that I wouldn't snap. She was staring at me so hard that it was easy to find her face. She shook her head because she knew what I was thinking. Her face said, "Please, Tionne. Don't." She knew I was about to go off right there in front of everyone. I took a deep breath and turned back to my microphone. "So," I said and continued the ceremony. It almost took Jesus himself to come down and stop me from cussing her out, but my mom's face was priceless. It was just enough to hold me back.

At the after-party, Prince came over to me. He was a funny guy. He talked a little bit like a robot, always with a deadpan voice. "You made me laugh," he said. "You're so funny. You wanted to whoop her ass."

"Yeah," I replied. "You think?"

I didn't care much for Aretha after that. But it was amazing that we were rolling with the big league now. We met

Michael Jackson, and he once told L. A. that I was his favorite member of TLC. L. A. respected my opinions about music back then, and I encouraged him to sign Outkast and Young-BloodZ. I gave him advice about some of his other artists, like Pink, for example. But I don't think she even knows that. L. A.'s brother originally wasn't going to check out Outkast, but I told him, "You're going to miss out. These guys are all that and then some." I called him at 1:00 a.m. to come down to the studio and hear them. He showed and ended up giving them a deal. I'd come a long way from being the kid dancing at Jelly Bean's every weekend. I was in it now.

It sounds like a lot of excitement and fame and shimmer. But it wasn't all great. Behind the curtain, TLC was dead broke. By the summer of 1995, as we unveiled "Waterfalls," we'd sold over 15 million albums. That made up over $75 million in album sales for the label, and TLC had literally nothing to show for it.

Here's how that's possible: For each album we sold, TLC got seven points (aka our royalty percentage out of 100), which equates to 56 cents. That was split between the three of us. Then we owed taxes. We owed a percentage to Pebbles, still, a percentage to LaFace and Arista, a payment to our accountant, and a payment to our lawyer. Each member of the band owed LaFace $100,000 and Pebbitone $50,000, thanks to our contracts with both companies. The amount of money we owed people seemed endless. So after all of the bills, in both 1993 and 1994, Lisa, Chilli, and I took home only $50,000 each. We were insanely low on the totem pole even though we were the artist. We were the ones out there working our asses off and touring and promoting the music to make it sell.

There was just no money. It was so messed up. I was living in a nice condo in Atlanta, and I couldn't even pay to keep my lights on. We had the No. 1 record in America, and we were the biggest girl group in the world, and we couldn't pay for anything. People expected us to have fancy cars and other glamorous things. But if you buy big shit, you have to be able to pay it off so you can keep it. Some of the labels's assistants had better cars than we did.

We were out of options. We were angry, and we needed to get control of the band's finances. I want to be really clear: We never said Pebbles stole from us. She was supposed to renegotiate our album contract after our first album dropped, but she didn't. That's standard practice in this industry. You always renegotiate the terms after a successful release. That was one of the main reasons we fired her. She did unfair business. We made more money as we became a bigger group, but we were stuck with the same low percentages. Her cut was supposed to change. In 5 years, we'd received 1 percent of $175 million worth of revenue from TLC. It just wasn't right.

Most people know the story of how we held Arista up at gunpoint to ask for our money. While we were in New York after *CrazySexyCool* came out, Lisa gathered up some of her crew from the diversion center. She had a plan. We'd asked L. A. for our money, and he said Clive had it. Okay, then we'd ask Clive.

Lisa was the ringleader, helping put it all together. Lisa had LaFace rent her a car to drive some girls from the diversion center and their guns up to New York. We always had this same limo driver when we went to New York City. He had a crush on me, and always left stuffed animals and flowers in the backseat. He was the getaway car for this escapade. He waited outside as we all marched into the Arista office and held everybody hostage. We never touched any of the guns—it was just the girls Lisa had met in the diversion center. There were eight or nine of us who barged in. Puffy was in a meeting when we arrived, and he called L. A. and some other folks to say we were wilding out after we politely asked him to leave his meeting with Clive.

"Yo," Puffy said on the phone to L. A. "Your girls up here mad buggin' yo."

"Sorry, but we gotta handle this," we told him.

We confronted Clive in his office while the rest of the girls went through the building taking down all the plaques with our name on it. To this day, you can find those plaques on eBay because we handed them out to whoever wanted them. We went down to the projects in Atlanta and just tossed out TLC plaques.

In the press, Clive had to shut it down quickly. The next day one of the newspapers in New York printed a story that we'd shown up at the label with all-male bodyguards, which we hadn't. And he didn't have a real answer for us. He was really talking in circles, something about our contracts. I wouldn't tell anyone to do what we did. It worked out okay for us—we didn't go to jail—but it wasn't ideal.

The truth is, you live and learn in the music business. It's a process. Knowledge is everything. You have to seek out information so you don't sell yourself short. You have to educate yourself, which we didn't know when we first started. We got swept up in the whirlwind and didn't realize we needed to advocate for ourselves as businesswomen. If you're smart, you figure that out fast, especially if you want longevity in this business!

In the end, our lawyer, David Bisbee, recommended bankruptcy to deal with our financial woes. Afterward, we'd have to renegotiate our recording contracts. On July 3, 1995, TLC filed for Chapter 11 bankruptcy. It was our best hope. It took months to resolve. Our lawsuit against LaFace, which we also filed, lasted for over a year. We had to just keep touring and being TLC until it was settled. Filing the paperwork it involved cost us each $15,000—a sum none of us had. Lisa asked Andre for the money (she'd reconciled with him after getting out of rehab), and thankfully he let us borrow it. We couldn't even afford to go broke on our own. We paid him back once we got back on our feet, but it was humiliating. It made me feel like I didn't have control over anything. The stress of everything made me sick, too. I kept having sickle cell flare-ups whenever something felt tense, which was all the time.

The record label flew us out to Los Angeles for the Grammys in early 1996. We'd gotten six nominations. It was a hell of a week. They put us up in the Four Seasons in Beverly Hills, and it felt like things escalated every single day we were there. There was this fancy jewelry store in the hotel lobby, with diamond necklaces and everything. We were still really furious at the label for low-balling us on our money, so we told our whole crew—the hairstylists, dancers, assistants, everyone—to go by the gift shop and charge whatever they wanted. We said, "Go get a diamond and charge it to our rooms." Our room charges went on the LaFace credit card. We racked up a $250,000 tab at the hotel, including $22,000 in that gift shop. Was it irresponsible? Maybe, but we were so unhappy and felt so slighted.

The first night in Los Angeles we wanted to go out to a club. When we got there, they refused to let us in because no one had ID.

"Fuck ID," Lisa said. "My face is my motherfucking ID!" It was embarrassing and hilarious at the same time. I was worried because Lisa was still on probation. We didn't need her getting into any trouble. She'd promised not to, but that promise clearly wasn't holding. She'd brought along her cousins Shere and Tangi and some friends from the diversion center again. Shere amped things up.

"My face is my ID," Lisa said again, pointing.

"Yeah," Shere said. "We're TLC!" Not only did the security at the club not let us in, but they removed us from the premises. The next night we tried a different club. As we pulled up, I saw Lisa on the street cussing out Shere and blocking traffic. Instead of parking, she'd jumped out of the car and left Shere inside crying. Shere sounded like a dying hyena and a baboon combined. Julie, our friend and stylist, and I convinced Lisa to park the car and unblock the road so people would stop honking at us. We went inside the club, and while we were sitting at our table, Shere kept trying to start fights with everyone around us.

"We'll fuck you up," she said. "That's TLC. Left Eye and T-Boz." She added, "We from Philly. See that white girl Julie? She'll kick yo ass, too."

We had nothing to do with it. She was getting us into trouble. She had a big mouth, and this wasn't the time.

I tried to stay positive. It was a crazy week, but maybe it could get better. I had done a job with Disney, and one morning I walked into the lobby of the Four Seasons to find a massive box of every single stuffed-animal dog from *101 Dalmatians*. It was as long as a car. It came up to my head. It was sitting there waiting for me, the two parents and all their puppies in a box, which was printed with black and white spots and tied with a red bow. It was the most amazing thing I'd ever seen. It was definitely the biggest gift I'd ever been given. I thought, "Things are looking up!"

I was mistaken, though. The real drama came the night of the Grammys, toward the end of the week. We won two awards, which was exciting, and performed "Waterfalls." It was fun and nothing seemed amiss, but things got dicey at the MCA Records after-party, which was back at our hotel. We'd stolen a bottle of Moët from the Sony party earlier in the evening for Lisa and her crew. I was outside, arguing with Dalvin about something dumb, when Julie ran out of the hotel doors.

"Lisa's on the bar," she exclaimed. "She's swinging at everyone!" I ran inside, Dalvin and Julie following me. Lisa was up there, wagging her fists and threatening the staff. Apparently the waitress had taken Lisa's bottle of Moët because Los Angeles bars had to close at 2:30 a.m. The waitress was rude and treated Lisa like a child, taking her bottle without any notice or permission. I tapped Lisa on the shoulder. She turned and didn't swing or yell. She just said, "She took my bottle! I told her it wasn't hers."

"We can get you another bottle," I said. I wanted to calm her down. I didn't know where I'd actually get another bottle from at the time.

"Fuck that," she replied. "I want that bottle."

Tangi chimed in. "Hell, yeah," she said. "Fuck that!"

"No," I said. "Lisa can't get in trouble. Please don't rile her up." Tangi stepped back. We had to keep Lisa out of jail. She probably wasn't supposed to be drinking since she was on probation, but it didn't occur to me at the time. We just needed to get her out of there in one piece. The staff started shutting down the party as we coerced Lisa off the bar. They called the cops and the party was shut down. They didn't arrest anyone because we promised to take care of Lisa. It took almost an hour and a half to do so. Lisa was so serious about that bottle of Moët. The hotel agreed to give her another bottle in the morning as long as Lisa kept the peace. They said they had to take all of the liquor out of her hotel room until the next day, too.

Finally, Jessica and I got Lisa into the lobby. Everything seemed fine. But then came Andre. He was slap-ass drunk, too.

"Baby, what happened?" he asked Lisa. Just what we needed, Andre here to stir things up. Lisa started getting all amped again.

"Dre," Jessica said. "We've got this."

"They're talking about taking her to jail," Jessica added. "We have to shut this down. She'll get her bottle back tomorrow. We just have to get her to her room."

He got her to calm down again, and we escorted Lisa to the elevators. Suddenly, out of nowhere, she started screaming and smacked her palms against the elevator doors. I don't know what happened—or why.

"No!" Lisa shrieked. "I'm not going up there!" She was yelling and taking off her clothes, right there in the elevator. She was about to get butt-naked. I couldn't take it. I threw up my hands.

"Jessica," I said, "you deal with it. If she goes to jail, I'm done." I didn't know what else to say. Lisa and Andre started arguing, and she was too drunk to reason with. I was so frustrated by it all. I left. Later I found out that Andre and Lisa, wearing only her drawers, had grabbed her belongings out of the room and left in a car and went back to Andre's hotel. She just bolted. It was a fitting end to a horrible week. And just imagine if cell phone videos and social media and TMZ had existed back then. But I will always admit that she kept things interesting and whether it was good or bad, I'd take her just like she was.

The bankruptcy was finally settled in April of 1996, and our lawsuit against LaFace that November. The settlement released us from all contractual obligations with Pebbitone, so we were now completely free of Pebbles. We would remain on LaFace. All of it was watched really closely by the music industry. It was a big deal to see a hugely successful act go broke because of bad contracts. We were leading by example, even if we didn't want to be the poster child for this. A lot of people saw what happened to us, and I hope it made young artists reconsider how to do their business. And I hope it made record label executives aware that it's not okay to take advantage of musicians. We were just glad it was over. We wanted to go back to being performers, instead of the subjects of news articles. It was time to move forward, both as a band and as people.

CHAPTER 6

The Truth

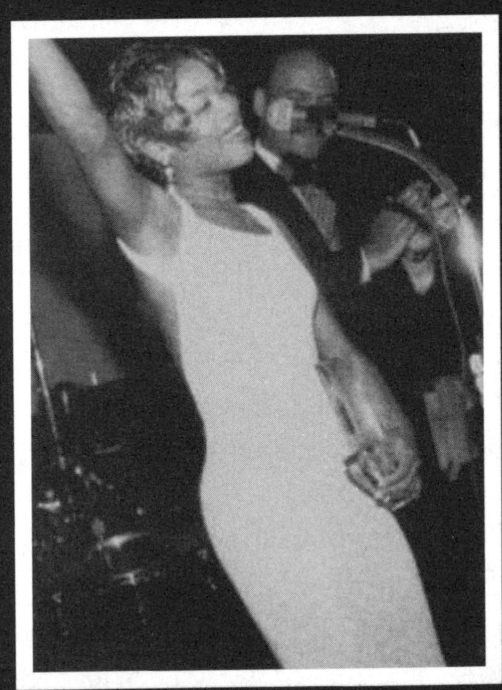

In the mid-'90s there were a lot of rumors flying around about celebrities and AIDS. Freddie Mercury had died of the disease in 1991, then Arthur Ashe. If a famous person got sick in public, it was assumed that's what they had. In the spring of 1995, rapper Eazy-E died from complications of AIDS, only a month after being diagnosed. It was a big deal in the press and made a lot of headlines.

Everyone was talking about it and trying to figure out if anyone else famous was sick. I was in and out of hospitals a lot—although most people didn't know why—and every time I went in, aching from the pain of my sickle cell disease, I'd hear people muttering to each other. They'd ask, "Does she have any symptoms?" They meant, "Does she have AIDS?"

At one of our shows, I collapsed on the side of the stage after we finished performing, and I left the venue in an ambulance. The press and our fans got wind that something was going on, and everyone made it into this big dramatic thing. Rumors started to spread. I'd met Eazy-E, but we'd never really hung out. We'd just acknowledged each other in passing. Still, there was speculation that I'd gotten AIDS from him before he died. It was the craziest thing, but everybody believed it. They wanted to believe it.

I could feel people whispering about me, assuming they knew what was going on with my body. This was before social media and rumors felt more substantial. It was harder for them to spread, so any that did had real force behind them. And this was one dumb rumor. It was people being ignorant, which I can't stand. But it all made me reconsider why I was being silent about my disease. I wanted to kill these ridiculous rumors, but I also wondered if there was any actual reason to keep hiding.

The pressure built. During one hospital visit, while we were out on tour, people who worked in the hospital made excuses to come into my room. Everybody kept coming in, pretending to do things like empty the garbage, just so they could see for real if I had AIDS. One guy even came in, opened a cupboard, found nothing, and left. I'd hear them asking one another, "Does she have any lesions?" Jessica got so fed up she cussed them out. And that's saying a lot, because Jessica didn't curse. Jessica is the only person outside of my family who would sit with me in the hospital. She cared about me as a person, not for what I could bring to the table. I will always love her for that!

"She's here because she needs help," Jessica shouted. It was stupid. Even if I did have AIDS, they'd still have to help me.

They all scurried away, probably to gossip somewhere else. They were ignorant. They associated me with the wrong disease. At the end of the day, it didn't matter what I had—sickle cell, AIDS, lupus, whatever—I was a person in the hospital. And instead of helping me, these people were being nosy and gossiping, completely ignoring my pain.

I wasn't certain I was ready to come out with it directly, though. I wasn't sure how to do it, even if I was ready. I didn't want to feel pitied. I got a call from a woman named Linda Anderson, who was running the Sickle Cell Disease Association of America. She'd heard from someone she knew that I had sickle cell. She asked if I wanted to be their new spokesperson.

"This could be a really good partnership," she said. "We could utilize you in a lot of positive ways."

It shifted my idea of what it would mean to be honest about my sickle cell disease. I could use it to raise awareness and hope. I could help to find a cure and teach people about the possibilities of alternative medicine. It didn't have to be about anybody feeling sorry for me.

So I said, "Okay, I'll do it."

On October 10th 1996, I threw a party at Liquid nightclub in Miami to announce that I was the new spokesperson for the Sickle Cell Disease Association of America—and to finally admit my own struggle with the disease. Everybody likes a party, and I wanted it to feel like a celebration. At the time, I was the youngest person—and the first woman and actual celebrity with the disease—to represent sickle cell and the foundation, and it felt like a really big deal.

Lisa and Chilli didn't show up for whatever reason. Who knows why. My mama was there, standing by my side like always, and the club was packed with close friends and family. Lots of press came, and I gave a short speech to announce my involvement with the cause. I just wanted to say my thing and let everyone get back to partying. They presented me with an award for my efforts, and after I spoke, She's the Man, a rock band I was managing, performed for the crowd. It was a hit. It made me so happy that I'd agreed to join up with SCDAA.

The next day *Entertainment Tonight* aired a segment on the party, revealing my secret to the public and to all our fans. No more speculation, no more rumors. I'd shut it all down and the truth was out. All that weight I'd been hauling around for decades had been lifted. I was free.

There's a legitimate liberation that comes from a confession, whether it's telling the truth about your disease to the world or just admitting something to yourself. Once you're no longer afraid of speaking the words, once it's all out there, there's a rush of freedom. It makes you wonder why you've held on to your secret for so long in the first place. I'm not defined by my sickle cell—I've never thought that. It's not who I am, even if the disease trails me wherever I go. Facing your fears and being honest with yourself is one of the hardest things you can do. But admitting to it let me become more myself, which is a very powerful thing. I could go forward into the world with one less thing to worry about.

When I first came out with the disease, I was 26, not yet correctly diagnosed, even after all these years. The doctors didn't really know what was going on with my body. They knew it was some type of sickle cell, they knew I was in pain, and that I had all of the symptoms every other sickler had—except for the physical characteristics. But there was no exact definition for it. They'd always told me I had a rare type of the disease that doesn't actually exist—sickle cell anemia and allegetic arthritis. If you Google that, it doesn't come up. After I'd started working with the Sickle Cell Disease Association, this guy named Phil Oliver started calling me. He worked for the Sickle Cell Foundation of Georgia, and he was determined to fix me—or at least to try to control my disease.

"I can help you," he said. "I've got some holistic methods."

I kept thinking, "Who is this psycho who keeps chasing me down?" But he was so persistent. One day he called and I couldn't help but give in. "Okay, fine," I said. "Help me."

After we spoke, I found out how knowledgeable Phil really was about sickle cell and realized he could actually help me feel better. He suggested acupuncture and a series of holistic remedies, so I went to see a Chinese herbalist named Dr. Lee, who had an office in Chinatown in Atlanta. Phil claimed he knew exactly what type of sickle cell I had. He was convinced. He pricked my finger right there in the lobby of Dr. Lee's office and tested it with a little kit he carried around.

"Yep," he said. "I knew it."

Phil instructed me to make an appointment with a doctor named Dr. Kenneth Braunstein, who was also based in Atlanta. My mama came with me to his office. I was sure this was going to be yet another idiot doctor who had no idea what was going on. I also thought he was going to be an asshole because the first thing he said to me was "No cell phones in this office."

I turned to my mama and said, "He's going to be mean."

"Give him a chance," she responded, patiently.

Dr. Braunstein took some blood, checked it, and came back into the room.

"You have sickle-thal with arthritis, which is sickle cell type SC mixed with beta-thalassemia," he said. It was a real mouthful. And it was the exact same thing Phil had said. I didn't entirely know what it meant, but Dr. Braunstein seemed very certain. This was it, not whatever other random diagnoses I'd been given since I was 7 years old.

It was an enormous relief to have a legitimate term for all I'd endured. I now knew what type I had so I could start trying to fix myself—if not completely heal myself—and I could make the best of it. It came after a lifetime of dealing with doctors who knew nothing or who had God complexes. A lot of them never knew what they were talking about, but couldn't bring themselves to admit it.

There was another wave of relief knowing, too, that I had found a doctor who actually cared. Dr. Braunstein was known for working with a lot of sicklers, who are especially prominent in the South. I could now walk into a hospital and say exactly what type of sickle cell disease I had, and they'd know better how to treat it—or so I thought. There was a real name for what I'd been feeling for decades.

After that, I began to understand sickle cell better. I knew how it affected me personally and how it could affect other people with the disease. I read a lot and asked questions. My type was rare—so rare that I didn't exhibit most of the physical characteristics typically common to most sickle cell patients. My external symptoms are dark circles or bags under my eyes, pink lips, and a pale face. Mine aren't permanent or everyday, like other patients' can be. You can tell when I'm tired or sick through my eyes. My mama can look at me and know I'm about to get sick, but I don't always show those traits. In fact, most of the time I didn't look sick at all, even though my symptoms on the inside are just as bad as any other sickle cell patient.

Dr. Braunstein did a case study on me after he became my doctor. He wasn't trying to experiment on me or make any guesses. He didn't want me to feel like a guinea pig or a lab rat, which a lot of doctors do. A lot of those guys do what I like to call guesstimating. They just hope they get some of it right. It always pisses me off when they don't know what's wrong and they refuse to admit it. If you don't know, just say you don't know. But even though I liked Dr. Braunstein, and even though I knew he cared, it didn't mean that I suddenly trusted all doctors. I still don't. But this was a huge step, just like admitting my disease to the world was a big step. No doctor has ever been there for me like Dr. B. We've become so close over the years, and I trust him with all of my health issues. I call him about medical issues that are not in his field, even if it's about a stubbed toe.

At the time, I wasn't sure how much my public admission helped anyone. I didn't know if me having the disease made other people feel better about having it, too. But I know now that it has. TLC has always tried to be a force of positivity and social awareness in the world, both as a group and as individuals. We aren't some pop band who makes music just to make music; we've always had a message. I knew my own experience could be an opportunity to help raise awareness and money for the disease, but it's only been in more recent years that I've seen just how much my own struggle has touched our fans personally.

People can be pretty self-involved. Some think only about their own stories, not about the stories around them. I'd always worried about what people would think of me if they knew I was sick. I didn't want the pity or the looks. But this was bigger than me. I could talk the talk, but I had to walk it, too. It was more important to push past my fears and help others than it was to sit there and be scared. I thought, "What am I here to do? Why did God put me on this Earth?

Why did he allow me to get through things that others didn't?"

I thought a lot about sickness. Not just my sickness, but the way all people deal with getting ill. It comes into all our lives, in some way or another.

In 1997 I started to see how illness can impact the people you love. My grandma Velma, who was still living in Des Moines at the time, started seeing her health decline. Her hips had deteriorated, and both of them had to be replaced. My mama used to fly back and forth from Atlanta to Des Moines to take care of her and help her with the surgeries. I'd always promised her that once I found success and earned some money, I'd buy her a place in Atlanta. It was now time to make good on my promise, especially since she'd been in pain for the past few years.

"It'd be easier if Grandma just lived here with you," I told my mama. She agreed.

My grandma was a stubborn lady. She'd been in Des Moines her whole life, and I wasn't sure if she'd leave Iowa. She was in her early eighties, and she had a community there. But I had to do what was right for her, and now I could afford to make it happen.

I built a house for my mom in Jonesboro, a small town outside of Atlanta, in a nice country neighborhood on a golf course. It had a two-bedroom and two-bathroom apartment downstairs for my grandma, with its own kitchen, living room, dining room, and den. I convinced her to move to Atlanta.

"Look at this," I said, gesturing to the downstairs apartment. I had a very serious tone in my voice. "Grandma," I said, "we built this for you."

She could live like a queen *and* be near her family. It

made me really happy that she agreed. On Thanksgiving Day my grandma arrived in Atlanta for good. Her hips were feeling better and her physical therapy had gone well, and she was fine for several months. It seemed like everything would work out.

But in early 1998, my grandma got sick again. She had already survived breast cancer, and I thought those days were behind us. The doctors diagnosed her with uterine cancer that had spread into her lungs. Her health started to fade more. My mom took her to visit her loved ones for the last time because we didn't know what the future held. There was a big family dinner, but after that, her health got even worse. She was admitted to the hospital, where the doctors said there was nothing more they could do. They gave her a choice between going to hospice or going home, and she decided that if she was going to pass, it should be at home.

A nurse came in and trained my mama and my aunts to give my grandma her medicines through a feeding tube. It required a lot of care. It was very upsetting for the whole family. We worked in shifts taking care of her. She was our matriarch, the center of the family, and it was up to us to make sure she didn't suffer in her final days.

I couldn't be there as often as I liked. I had contractual obligations to TLC. We went into the studio to start working on our third album, *FanMail*, in April of 1998, and that became all too consuming. I went home to Mom's house as much as I could, and I sat with my grandma even after studio, no matter how tired I was. Sometimes I would even cancel studio sessions. I sat with her even if she was sleeping. She was a small woman, only about 5 feet 2 inches, but she was powerful, and she had an inner strength that she carried throughout her illness. She lost her hair during chemo and her weight dropped significantly. She became sensitive to smells and noise. I'd watch her and think how small and fragile she seemed.

I remember one visit very clearly. Grandma was on the couch, very quiet. She reminded me of a baby bird. She refused to wear her wig in the house, although sometimes she'd wear one outside if she was feeling better. She was 83 and there were no wrinkles on her face. I gazed at her and marveled at how beautiful she looked.

"Grandma," I said, "you're really pretty."

"Oh dear, you've got to be kidding me," she replied. She didn't seem to believe it.

"No, really," I said, "your face is flawless. It's so clear. It's so pretty." I added, "So what if you're smaller than you used to be?" I really meant it, and I think she could see that. It seemed to make her feel a little better. She and I had a special bond. I'd had IVs stuck in me my whole life. I knew what it felt like to be sick and to feel helpless in your own body. But for some reason, her illness seemed harder than my own.

"Your disease is so much worse than mine," I told her. "I don't think there's any comparison."

My grandma just shrugged. "Pain is pain," she said.

But I've always felt like pain isn't just pain for everyone. I go through a lot, and it may be worse than what some people deal with, but it's not comparable. Pain differs based on who you are. Pain is pain, but some is severe and some is light, and what is severe to someone else might be light to me. When you watch someone go through something, it can feel like the worst thing in the world. I've seen others have a cold and act like they're dying. They don't know anything worse. We all have a different pain threshold, which is something I've learned over the years as I've been sick and as I've watched other people get sick.

It was really tough to watch my grandma going through chemo, but she always stayed positive. There was always a smile on her face, and she wouldn't let anything bring her down or defeat her. I remember once asking her, "Are you going to give up or are you going to keep fighting?"

She smiled at me, as she always did. "What do you think?" she replied. "Of course I'm going to fight it, sweetie. I'm never going to give up."

She didn't, either. Not even when she got sicker and was confined to her bed. It taught me even more about dealing with illness. As I saw her inner strength, I realized that disease is only as powerful as you allow it to be. Even when your body is breaking down, your mind and your heart and your spirit can shine through. I realized that my own day-to-day problems felt insignificant. If she could push through, then so could I.

Just before Halloween, I got sick with the flu. I couldn't be around my grandma because her immune system was out of whack from all the chemo and medications. I stayed at my mama's house, but avoided contact with my grandma because she couldn't afford to catch my cold. Anyone with cancer shouldn't be around other germs. I sat in the living room and stared at her lying in her hospital bed from afar. We were in the midst of finishing *FanMail*, and I wanted her to be able to hear it. But she hadn't been able to focus in the past few weeks and couldn't listen to anything, especially not the new TLC album. She was in too much pain. In the middle of the night, on Halloween, someone woke me and said Grandma was breathing funny. We called the ambulance and took her to the hospital. Maybe there was something the doctors could do for her that we couldn't.

"There's nothing we can do," one of the doctors confirmed. "We just have to wait."

They said she would pass away within hours, but she didn't. So we waited. We sat in the hospital and waited by my grandma's side. She held on for so long—2 more weeks, to be exact. The doctors gave her pain meds through her IV, and she fell into a coma. I'll never forget the gurgling sound her body made in her last hours. I knew she could hear us because when we spoke to her, she would gurgle. That's how we knew her time was near. It was a response of some kind. I saw for myself that people in a coma can hear you.

A minister arrived and gave her last rites. My grandma had been right when she said she would fight until the very end. She woke momentarily from the coma and said, "Someone please let me out of here. I want to go home."

But she didn't ever go home. A few days later, I sat in the hospital lobby, watching TV, and my mom came to get me. It was time. Grandma had slipped back into the coma. We formed a circle around her and sang. One of the nurses started crying and told us she'd never heard a family sing to a dying loved one before. But we wanted Grandma to know we were there. She'd always loved to hear her children sing. We wanted to ease her journey into the other side. We wanted her to feel the love all around her as she left us. We sang

"Jesus Loves Me," one of her favorite songs, and waited. Her breathing grew shallow.

My mama took her hand. "Go ahead and rest," she told Grandma. "You can let go. It's okay."

My grandma took one long final deep breath and she was gone. I could feel her leaving. One moment she was there, and then she wasn't.

It was a hard time for me. I was just coming to grips with my own illness and finally having a legitimate diagnosis, and now I had to say goodbye to a woman who had helped to shape my life. The loss was profound. I ached inside. I regretted that she never got to hear *FanMail*, which we'd essentially finished by the time she died. I regretted that she wouldn't be there for the rest of my life and for the rest of my career, and she would never see me have the kids I hoped I'd have and grow older. I knew how close my own mom was to her mother, and seeing my mom in pain was hard. I saw what sickness could do to the human body and how much pain it could cause everyone around you. It made me want to fight harder, to empower myself even more. Pain is pain, my grandma had said, and it affects everyone in some way. I wanted to be stronger now. I wanted to push through my pain, like she had.

When I look back now, I think that God has spared my life because I am supposed to help people with my story. I can be a walking testimony of strength and power, and I can decide not to be afraid, just like my grandma.

Ten years ago I got small tattoos on my hands: a heart, because there's nothing stronger than the love in a mother's heart, and two butterfly wings. I've always associated my disease with butterflies—they start out ugly and cocooned, but later they grow and fly free and it's beautiful. I got the tattoos as a reminder, so I could look down at my hands any time I got upset, down, or scared. They remind me of the work my hands and my body has to do and why I am supposed to stay here. I've got people to inspire. I've got music to make. I've got things to do. I won't stop until one day I wake up and a doctor tells me, "Girl, you don't have cooties no more."

CHAPTER 7

The Battle Within

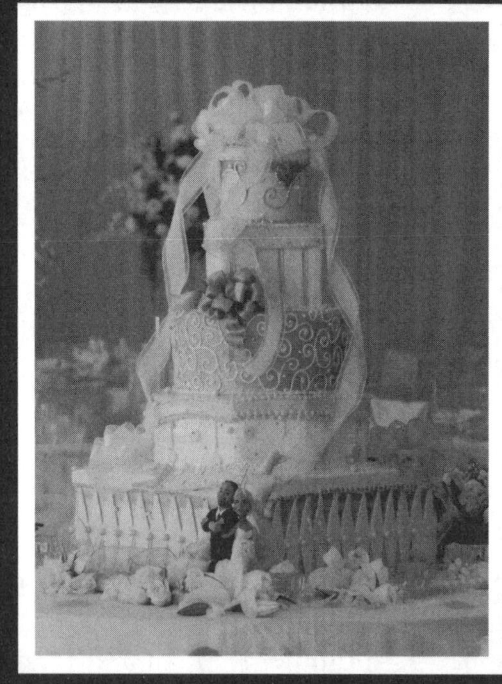

We rode high on the success of *CrazySexyCool*. But it was a lot of pressure, too. We knew we needed a follow-up album that was as good. I never try to outdo the last hit just to make more hits. Songs like "Waterfalls" are hard to come by, so every time you make an album, it's a lot of pressure. It doesn't get easier just because you know what you're doing or you've been in the studio before. You have to keep evolving and getting better every time.

One thing I always try to keep in the back of my head is to aim for an album like *Thriller*. It had nine consecutive hits, so I make that my goal. You want to get at least two or three hits on one album to make it worthwhile and to give it longevity.

As we started writing new music, there was tension in the band between me, Chilli, and Lisa. I could feel things slowly starting to crack around us. My perfect career was not as seamless as it appeared from the outside.

Lisa started talking badly about TLC but mostly about the people we were working with, to anyone who would listen. She talked to everyone but the people involved. If we ever sat down to talk to each other honestly, it had to be at the right time—but it was never the right time because Lisa's then-boyfriend was always in her ear. She had issues with Dallas, too, which she was vocal about.

"I wanna say something without saying too much," Lisa said on-camera at one point. "I'm just gonna be honest with everybody." She told the press that Dallas had charged us too much money to record some songs in the past. "So he might not be on the project," she added. "We've been fighting with Dallas for about 10 months." She always felt like she had to tell it like it was, no matter how it looked.

We needed to deliver this third album. It wasn't up for negotiation, and we didn't have time for this drama. We had the idea to make a collection of songs that was dedicated to our fans. It could be their album and their songs. Much of our fan mail never got answered, and a lot of fans were upset because they wanted us to reply back to them. We were never able to get around to each and every one of them. It wasn't like today with Twitter. These were actual letters. Usually you hire a company to reply to your fan mail on your behalf. We used to read as many as we could and reply to them ourselves, but that required more time than our schedule would allow. So the best way to give our thanks to the listeners was to put their names inside the CD jacket for the album. We called it *FanMail*. Lisa was always awesome with album titles, and she did it again here. Our art director had a photo of Naomi Campbell painted silver, and that picture inspired me to have us look like space cadets on our album cover.

Once again, it was me, Dallas, and Leslie together in the studio most of the time. LA Reid decided I should go to Minneapolis to record with Jimmy Jam and Terry Lewis, who were known for working with Janet Jackson and Prince. I was really excited. It felt like the opportunity of a lifetime. I was thrilled to walk into their studio, Flyte Tyme, where Janet and Prince had worked. I went 3 days earlier than Lisa and Chilli and met with Jimmy and Terry to discuss what sort of song I wanted to do. I'll always remember that day because Jimmy Jam taught me a technique I had never used before.

"Go into the recording booth," he said. "And hum or sing whatever comes to the top of your mind, no matter what it is." I went in as he played the beat. I sang whatever melodies I heard as he recorded it, and then the two of us picked which ones might be usable for the verse and hook. It felt really revelatory. We put words to the melodies and suddenly there was a song. It ended up being "I'm Good at Being Bad." I still use that technique. It's a different way to write music and it feels very open. I write songs other ways as well. It depends who I'm working with as to what technique is used, but this was a cool new way to write something.

The inspiration for the tracks on *FanMail* came from a lot of places. We wrote the music in a lot of different places and in different ways. For me, though, the most important song was "Unpretty." Writing it was almost an accident. I was in Los Angeles with Dalvin, who was still my boyfriend at the time. We were staying at the Montage, a fancy hotel in Beverly Hills. The skyline sparkled outside. I love skylines—they look like art created by God to me. It was beautiful, but I was sad. I'd just gotten out of the hospital and I was feeling really ugly.

There's this period of withdrawal you go through after being on all the medication, so you feel like you're not in control of your body. My nervous system was acting up. I was shaking, and having hot and cold flashes. I had bruises from all the IV attempts.

Dalvin didn't get it. We'd been together for a while and he'd seen me sick, but he never quite seemed to understand what I needed after a crisis. He never came to see me in the hospital, either. He said he didn't want to see me that way. It's not about how you feel, though. It's about how the person in the hospital feels. That night, in LA, he left to go out with some friends, and I shouldn't have had to tell him to stay there with me and keep me company. I don't think he would have stayed even if I'd asked, which hurt worse. So I sat in the hotel room, the lights dim, flipping through the TV channels. I paused on Ricki Lake's show. The topic of that night was men who abuse their wives. It was really dark. The women were so wounded and unhappy. You could see the pain in their eyes. I felt unhappy that night, too, but my hurt was nothing compared to these women. I really felt for them.

After the show ended, I turned off the TV and sat there for a long time. I thought about all the women who feel like they aren't good enough. All the women who feel too skinny or too fat, too tall or too short, or who feel unattractive in any way. I thought about how we all have something in common. We've all felt unpretty and not good enough to fit into society at some point. It's not only women, but men, too. It can be about our clothes or our appearance. We get bullied or teased in school, and everyone has some kind of complex about their looks. Where does that come from? How does that feeling get inside us? I think most of the time it's other people putting it there. Relationships can be amazing, but they can also have

Me at age 12

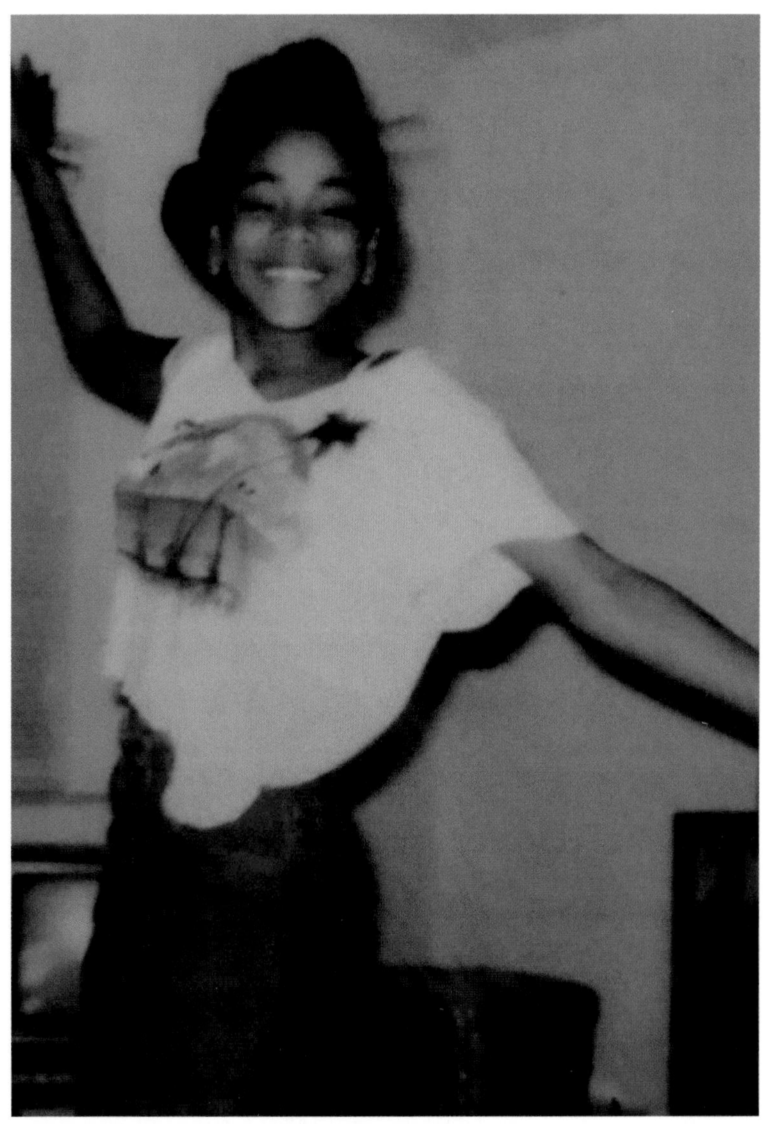

Top Left: 11th grade prom
Top Right: DeVyne Stephens, who encouraged me to be a choreographer, and me
Bottom: My Aunt Ressie and Cousin Donnie

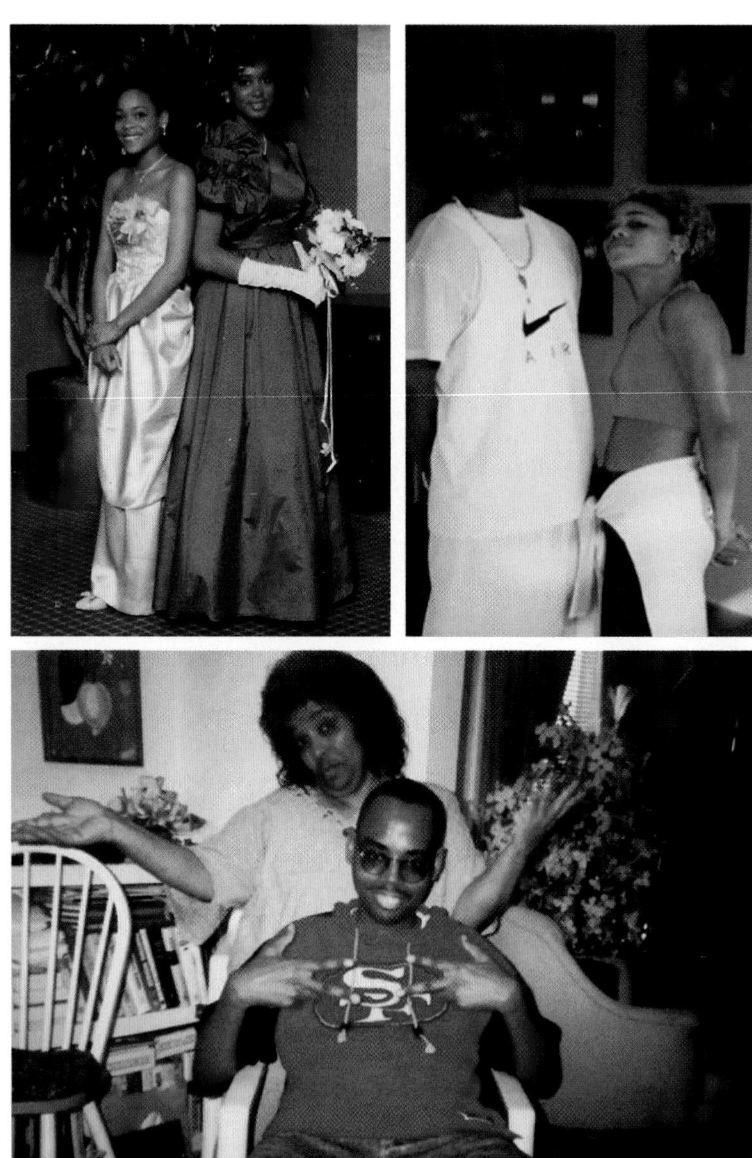

Top: My father, James, in his band, the Martinells.
Bottom Left: Me at age 3
Bottom Right: Me at the 2002 MTV Video Music Awards

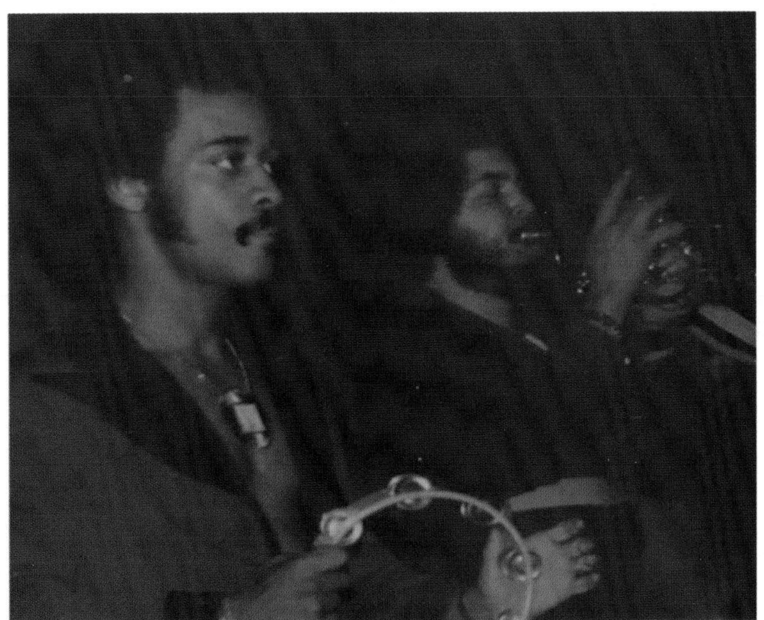

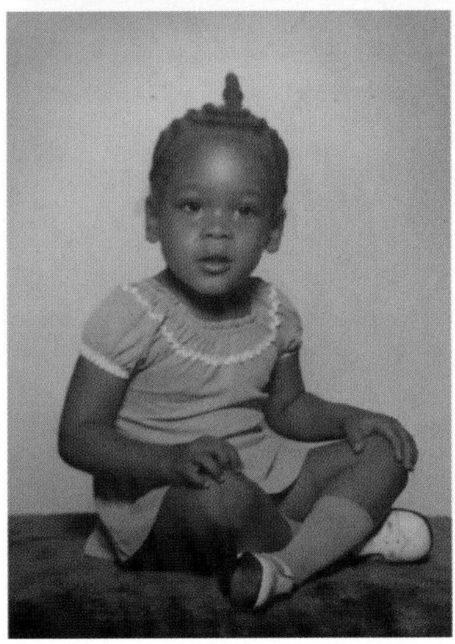

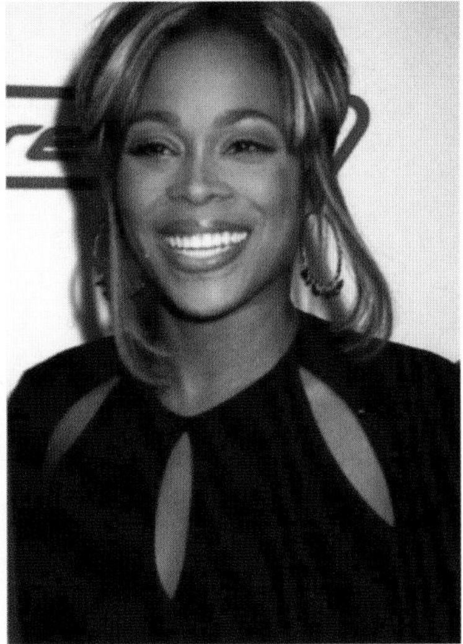

Top: Lisa and me in our Second Nature days
Bottom: Lisa after our food fight at Doppler Studios

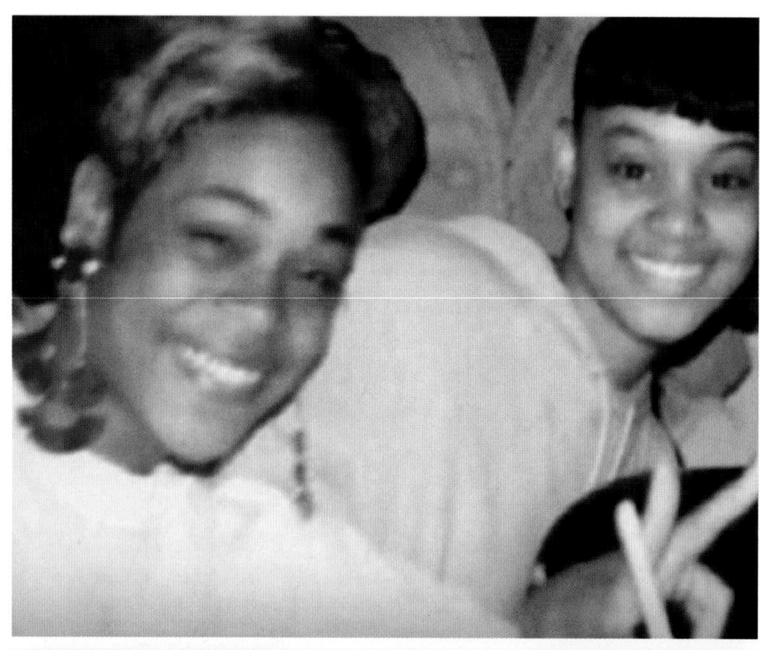

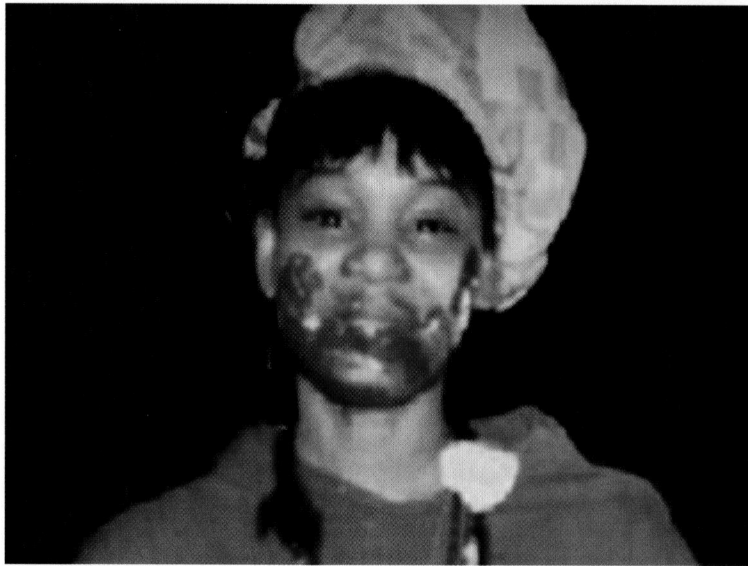

Top left: My mom
Top right: A rare photo of me in a dress!
Bottom: A photo shoot for *People* magazine after my brain surgery, showing I can still dance

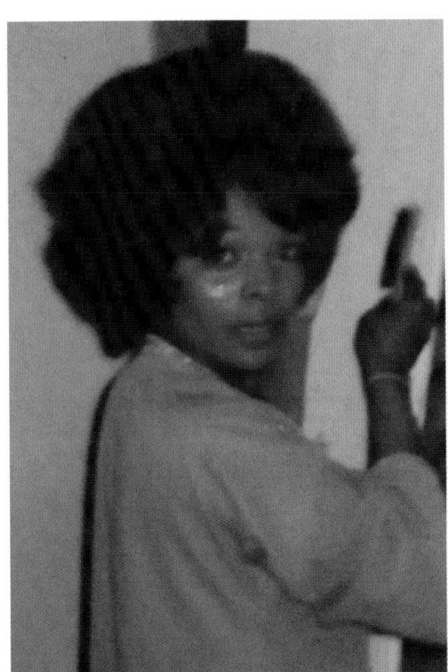

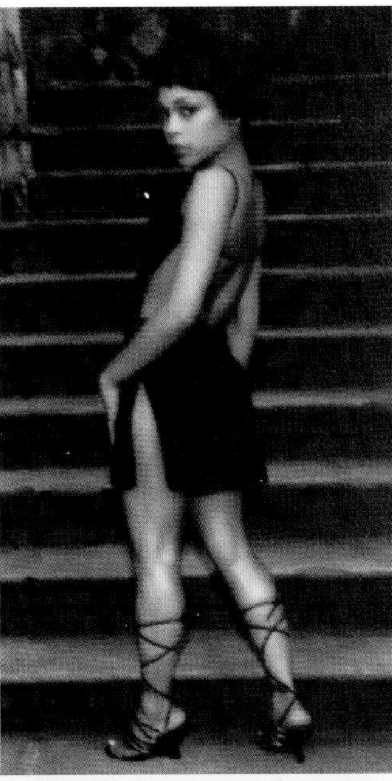

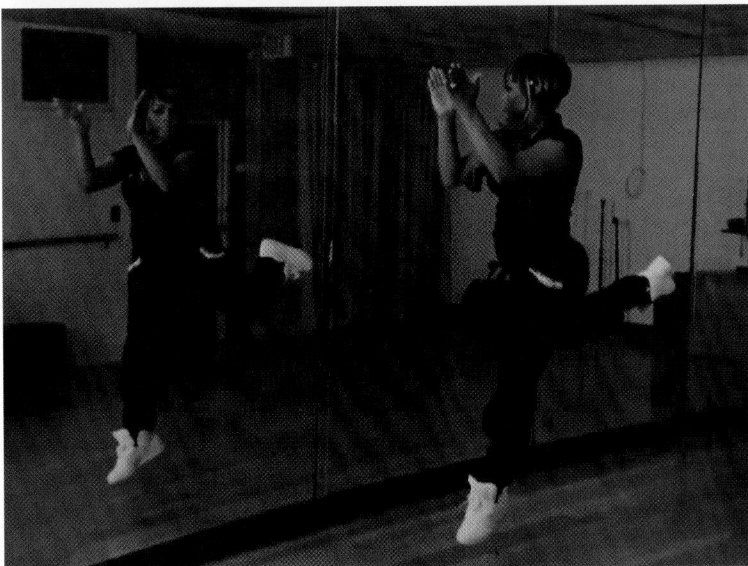

Shanti, Nechole, me, and Tae Tae

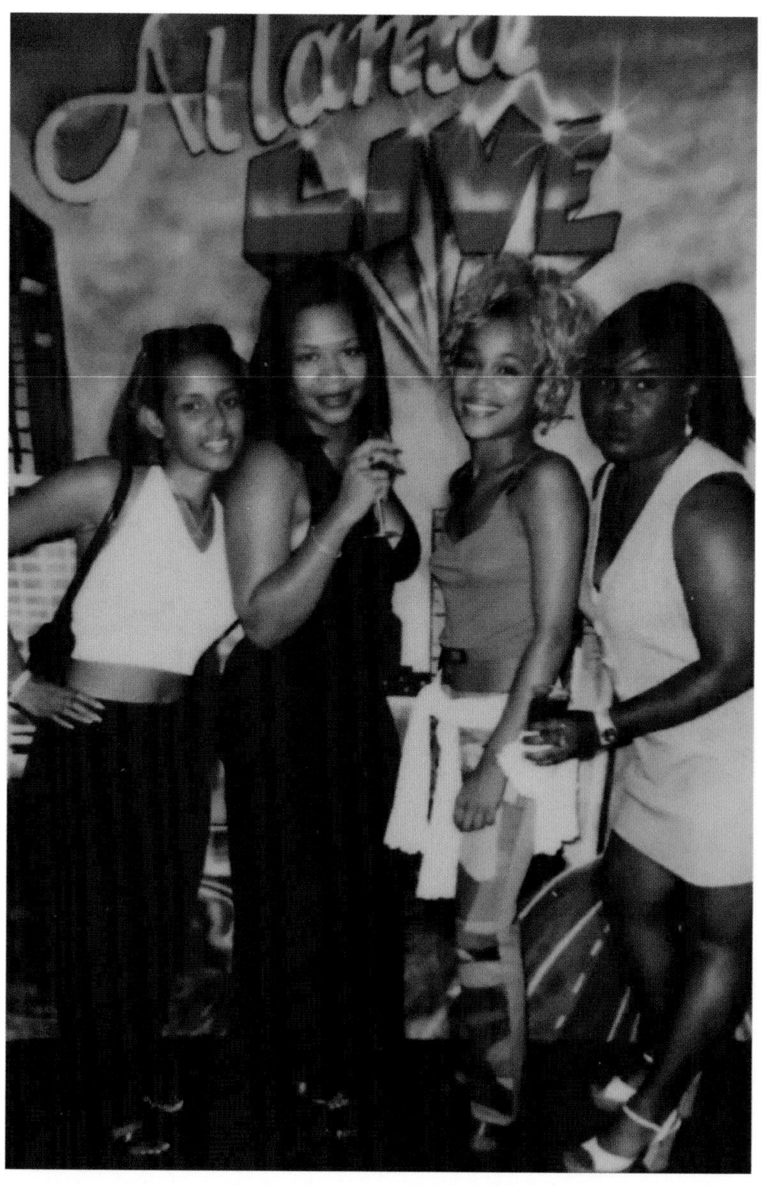

Chase and Chance (2 months)

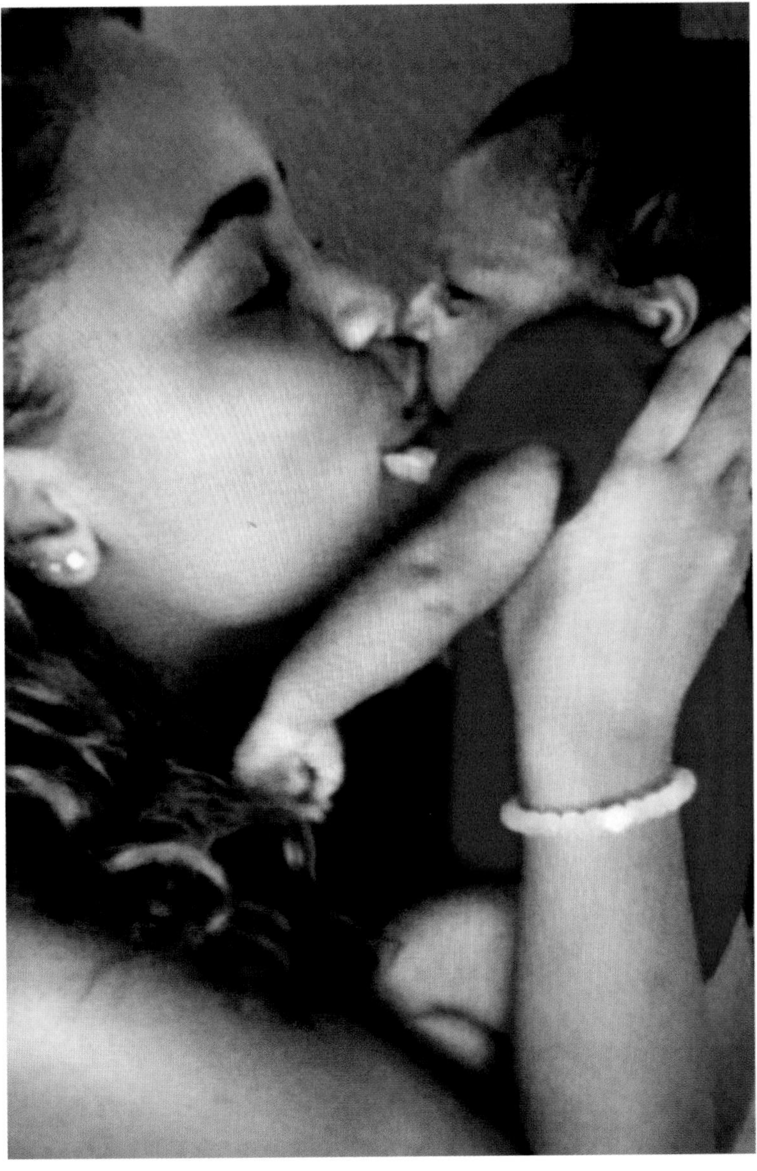

Top: TLC's Fanmail tour
Bottom: Legendary makeup artist Kevyn Aucoin and me

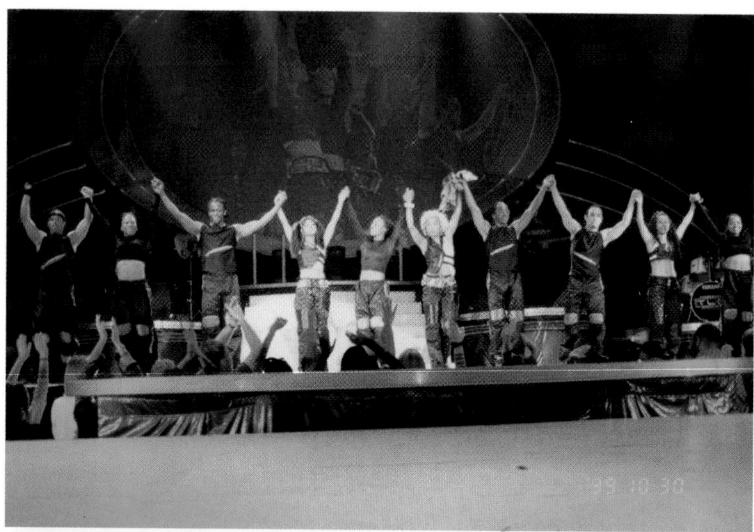

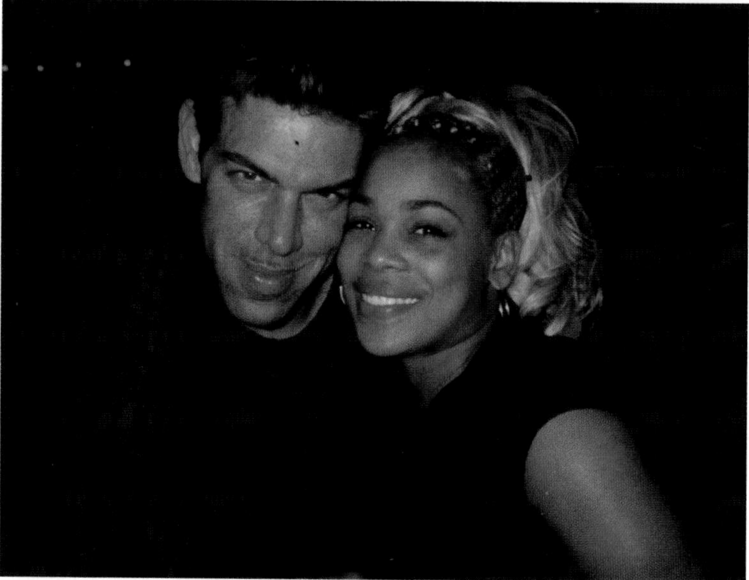

Top: Photo Shoot for *Vibe* magazine
Bottom (from left to right): Nechole, me, Yolonda, Gail, and Barb

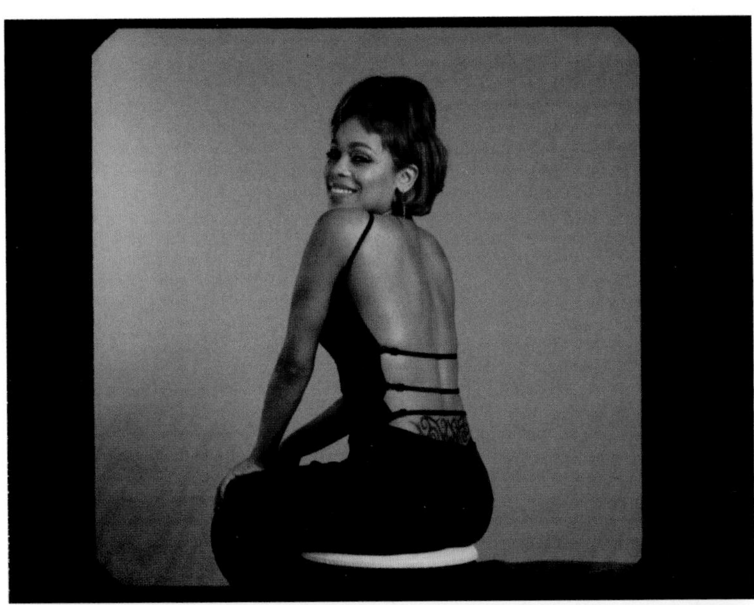

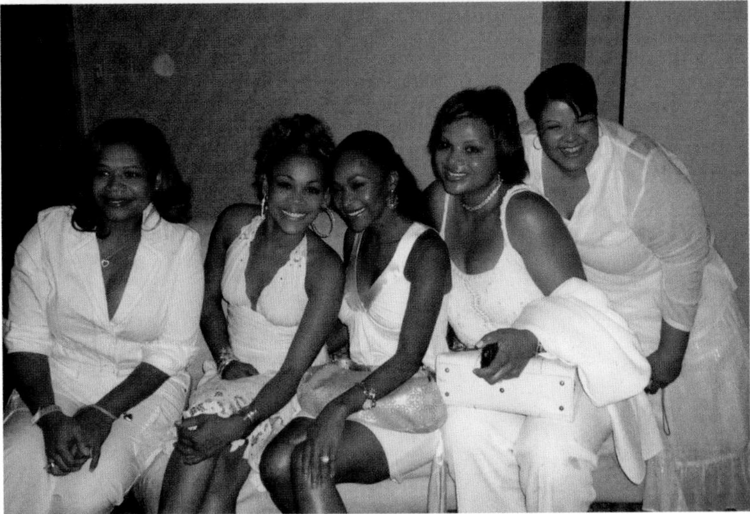

TLC at the 1996 Soul Train Awards

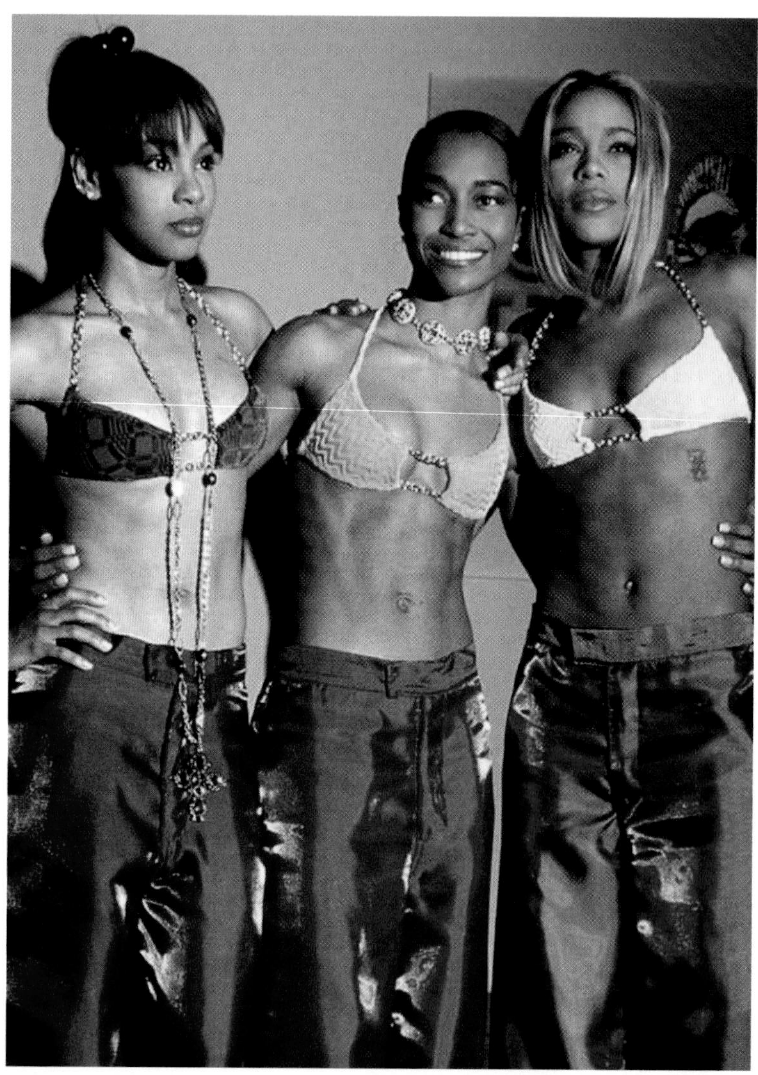

My wedding reception

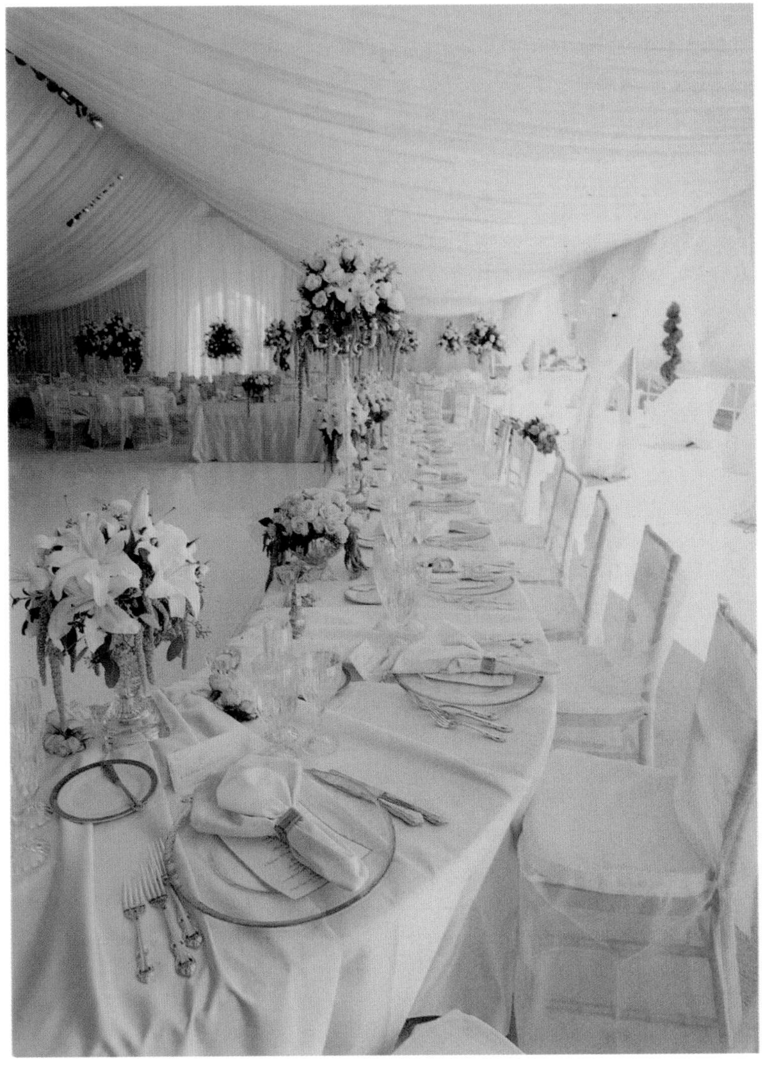

Top: Doing press for Chase's Closet at home
Bottom: On the set of *Belly*

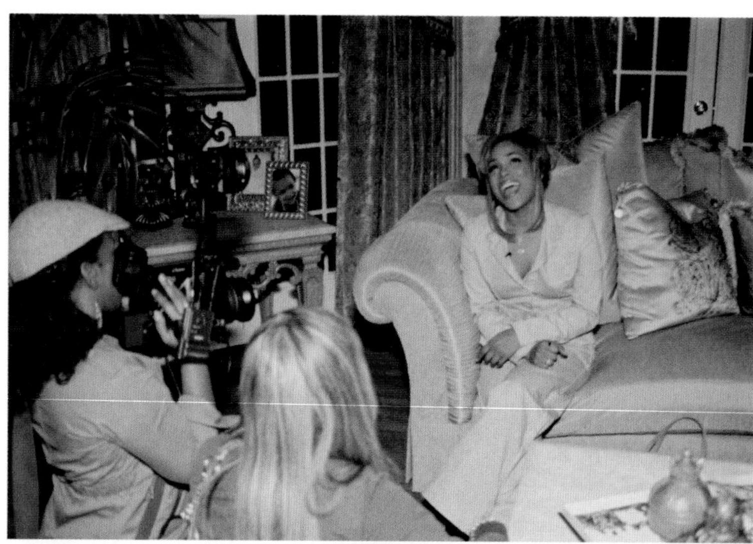

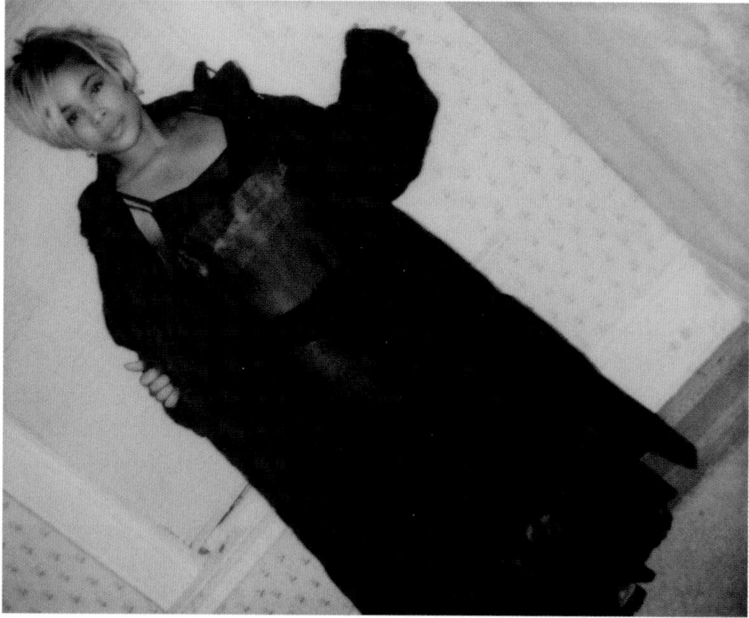

Top Left: In Barbados doing a BET Special (another rare moment of me in a dress!)
Top Right: Chase's first Halloween
Bottom: Chance's first birthday, giving mommy kisses

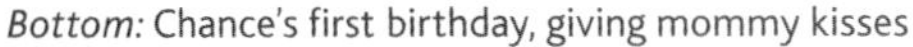

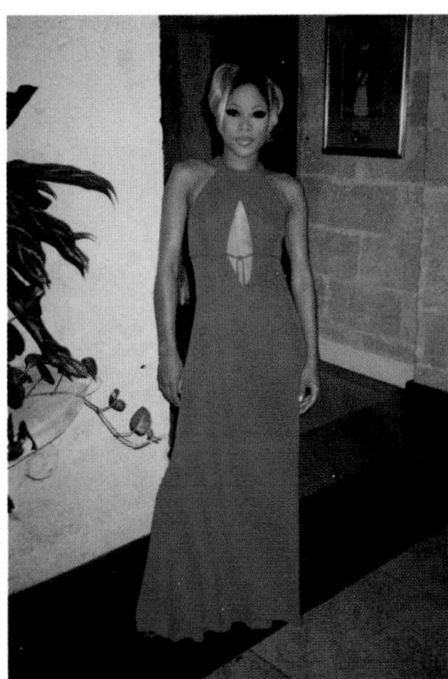

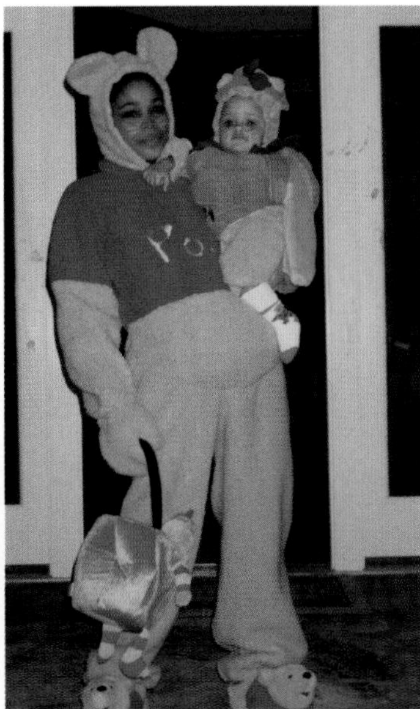

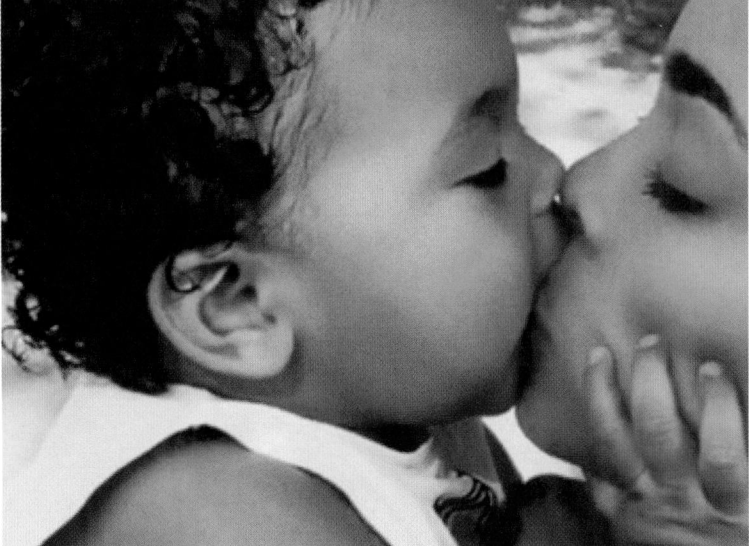

Top: My cousin Marde and me.
Bottom: Tara, my partner in running Chase's Closet, and me

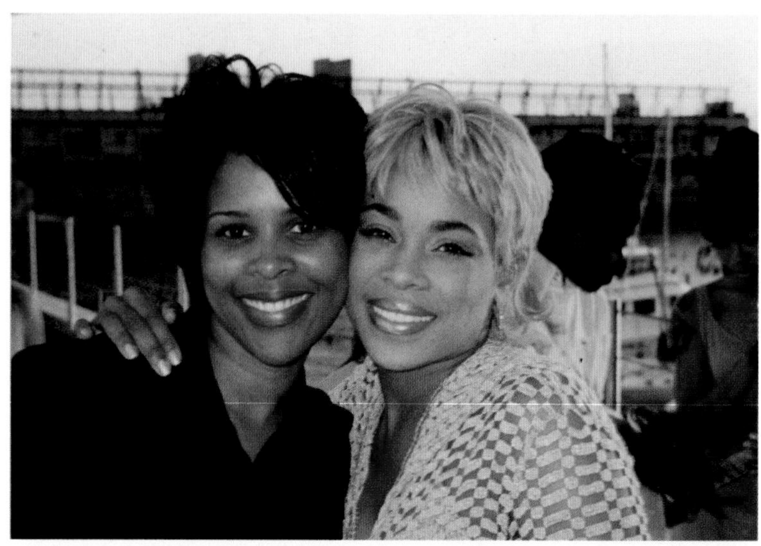

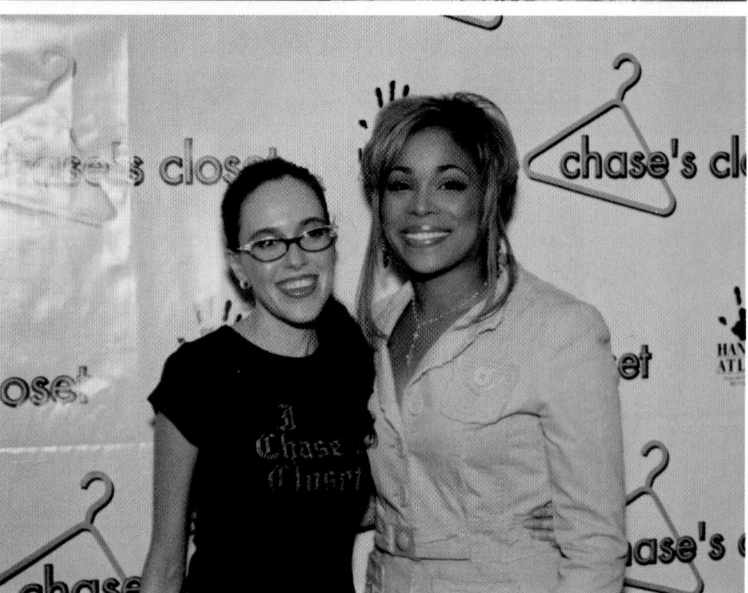

Top: Us with Billy Idol at Total Recall. This was our last performance with Lisa.
Bottom: TLC photo shoot in pants I designed—Lisa's uncle made them for us.

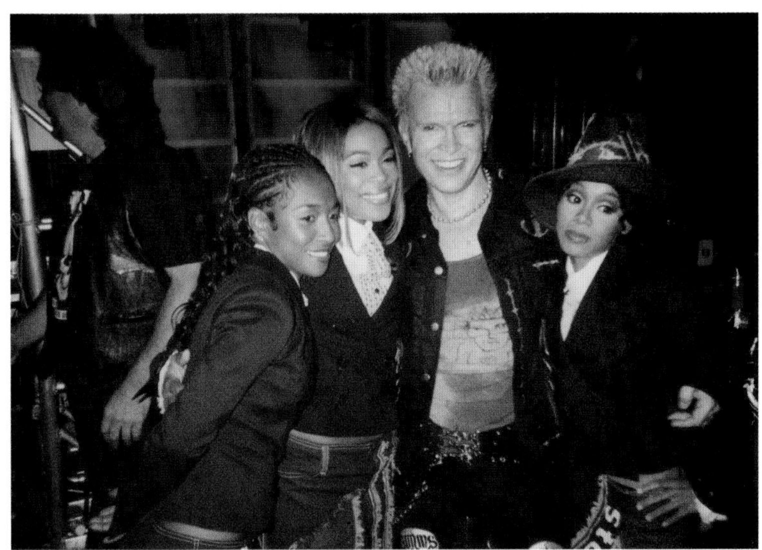

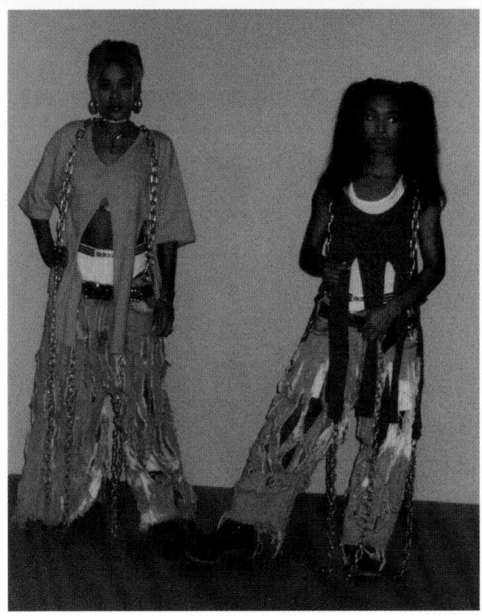

Chance and me

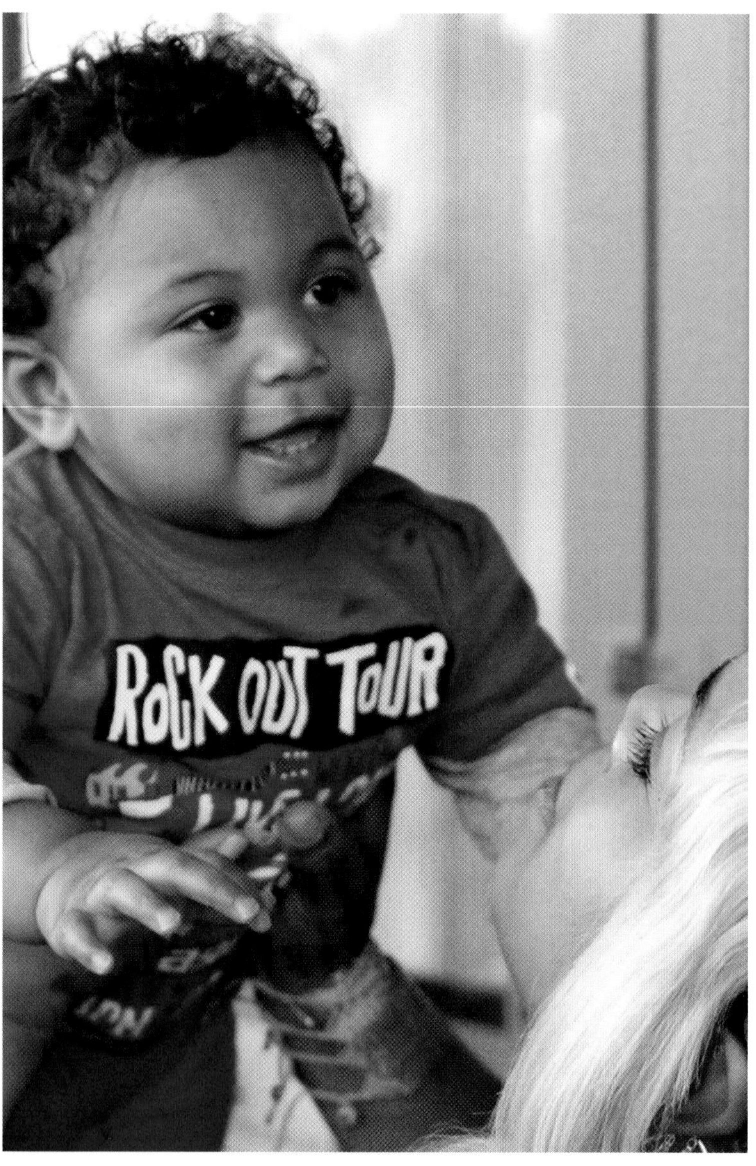

a negative side. Other people shouldn't have power over you and your emotions, but they do. They can put those bad feelings in your head and heart, and cause your pain to surface. We all have the possibility to make someone else feel unpretty.

I needed to do something with these emotions. That's the point of being an artist, right? You feel something and you have to get it out. I'd never written a poem before, but that seemed like a good way to channel these thoughts. I'd written songs and lyrics, of course, but poetry wasn't exactly my thing. Suddenly words were pouring out of me, pen onto paper. I had so much to say. I scribbled out lines, and within moments, there was a complete poem on the page before me. It was titled "Unpretty." More poems followed. Those became the foundation of a book I released in 1999, called *Thoughts*. It was poems and essays about my life, and it was dedicated to the fans who asked me for guidance in their own lives.

When I showed Dallas my writing, it became clear to us that "Unpretty" could become something more. Dallas and I transformed the poem into a song. He helped me put the lines into the form of musical art. It was a song most could relate to, so Lisa and Chilli really embraced it. It ended up becoming one of TLC's biggest songs, a track that I hope has helped fans around the world come to terms with who they are and how they look. I've had people stop me on the street to tell me how the song changed their life or how it kept them from committing suicide, which is deep. I aimed to help when I wrote the song, but I never thought it would be that powerful.

I've always struggled with my appearance and my weight. I'm like anyone else—I don't wake up feeling perfect every day, and being a celebrity doesn't change that. In fact, being photographed on red carpets and having your every move scrutinized can make it worse. It's not like I go around caring what people think on a daily basis, but during the times when I have a medical issue and I'm trying to heal, it can be really emotionally, physically, and mentally draining, let alone to have a camera in your face. And now with social media? Forget it. When I was a teenager, I was super skinny. I didn't have the big old butt you were supposed to have. Sometimes I layered two pairs of pants on top of each other, trying to fake like I was thicker. It seemed like all the guys liked thick girls, especially growing up in the South. Guys would call my friends "fine," but refer to me as "cute" or "pretty." I wanted to be fine, too. I obsessed over blemishes, and I felt awkward when I saw photos of myself with dark circles and bags under my eyes.

You always see yourself differently than others see you. And despite what you see in the magazines and on album covers, no one really looks that perfect. It takes airbrushing and Photoshop to make women look that slick and smooth. But there's no such thing. We all have a flaw or two. My friends would say "you have clear skin, no acne, and you don't have to wear makeup, so what are you tripping about?" But to me, my dark circles ruined everything. Later I found that it didn't stop me from getting boyfriends, and others didn't see them the way I did! And what is so funny is that when I get a compliment, it's usually about my eyes. So the thing I thought was my worst feature is my best to others. It's easy to look at images of celebrities and feel like you don't measure up. And we all feel like that—even the celebrities. That's what "Unpretty" is about. It's about all the times you've felt lesser than or that someone has made you feel like you're not good enough. It's meant to help those who hear it overcome their own self-doubt and insecurity. It's about finding the beauty within yourself.

The video for "Unpretty" was directed by Paul Hunter over the course of almost a week in Valencia, California. It was a pricey video—$1 million—but it was worth it. We wanted to tell a real story that viewers could relate to. It came out really beautifully. Seeing my original vision for the song come to fruition in a music video was meaningful to me, a dream come true.

By that time I had broken up with Dalvin. Things had been up and down with us for a few years, and it was finally time to go our separate ways. I remember the date of our breakup because it was the same day *The Players Club* came out. I went to see it with my really good friends Nechole and Tae Tae in Atlanta. Outside the theater, as we were leaving, I looked at the sky and said, "This looks like tornado weather."

"You've been watching too many *National Geographic* shows," Nechole said.

"I'm telling you," I said. "This is a tornado sky." After I got home, I realized I was right. Rain was pouring down. The door swung open, and I had to go outside in the rain and pull it back in. The phone went blank and the TV crackled. Suddenly the rain stopped, the lights went out, and everything went dead silent. My entire house shook.

"Lord," I said, "please don't let this be a tornado." Lights from the lightning were flashing everywhere in the house. My door blew open again. I ran to my basement in terror. I covered myself in Plexiglas. It turned out to be an F5 tornado, right there on the corner of my street. It took part of my roof off and knocked my tree down, but it left my house standing even as it destroyed the entire street behind my property. It was horrible. God spared me, and when I went upstairs, I paused and thought to myself, "Why am I bothering to be with people I'm unhappy with? This relationship with Dalvin is going nowhere. I need to get rid of people who are bringing me issues."

I called Dalvin. "This relationship isn't working," I told him. "I could have died in this tornado and I'm not happy with you."

That was that. I don't know if he ever really understood why we broke up, but I couldn't be unhappy any longer. Writing "Unpretty" had helped me see that, but it was a long time coming, and it took an actual tornado to blow him out of my life.

During the "Unpretty" video shoot, I was still single. I'd recently worked with Quincy Jones III, who is the son of Quincy Jones. He came down to the video shoot and brought an artist named Mack 10 with him. Mack, whom I call D'mon, was a rapper and also a part of Westside Connection with Ice Cube and WC. He had successful albums solo and with the group. I noticed immediately that he was cute.

"You got pretty eyebrows," D'mon told me while he was hanging out on set. I started laughing. What kind of compliment is that? But he had the gift of gab. After we wrapped shooting for the day, a bunch of us went out to dinner and he came along. He ended up paying for everyone. He got my number, and we'd talk daily on the phone after I got back to Atlanta. We hit it off really quickly. Eventually, he asked me out.

"Okay," I said. "But you have to fly me and my friend Nechole out to LA together." I needed backup. I wasn't going cross-country to hang out with this guy alone. To this day, I've never been on a date by myself. My rule is that you have to take me and my friends or family out until I see if I like you. As it turned out, I liked D'mon. We were together after that, and Mack 10 and T-Boz became a well-known celebrity couple for a while. He ended up being there for a lot of TLC's drama over the next few years.

"No Scrubs" was the other important song on *FanMail*. It was produced by Kevin "She'kspere" Briggs and written by former Xscape members Kandi Burruss and Tameka Cottle, and it felt perfect for us. I'm sure you know this, but for those who don't, a "scrub" is a guy who lives at home and does nothing with his life. He lives off his mother or his baby mama. He lies about material things. He's the loudest guy yelling out of the window of the Benz, but it ain't his Benz and he's in the passenger seat. He's always talking about what he wants, but he's also always sitting on his broke ass. We became famous for that term, and it's still popular. I still get guys coming up to me like, "I own this car! I'm no scrub."

The video for "No Scrubs" was directed by Hype Williams and shot in March of 1999. The concept was really futuristic, and the three of us had to climb up a ladder into this rotating metal box they'd built on a sound stage in Los Angeles. It was drilled closed and it was unique—in a weird kind of way. There wasn't enough oxygen, so they had a fan blowing, and we had to take breaks to catch our breath. We'd bang on the floor to get them to stop filming, and they'd unscrew the floor so we could stick our faces out to breathe. We danced while the box spun around, which looks a lot easier than it was. Videos are usually only fun after they're done being shot. They look great, but they're always a trial to do. It was worth it, though: We ended up winning the 1999 MTV Video Music Award for Best Group Video for "No Scrubs," beating out Backstreet Boys and NSYNC.

When I look back now, it's a miracle these videos even happened. The drama within the band had amped up so much that the press started speculating whether we were going to break up before the album even dropped. Lisa amped it up even more. We did a photo shoot and interview for *Vibe* magazine right before the album came out, and Lisa took it upon herself to stir things up. A week after our interview, she called the writer.

"I cannot stand 100 percent behind this TLC project and the music that is supposed to represent me," she told the reporter. "This will be my last interview until I can speak freely about the truth and present myself on my solo project." She had told me how she felt and said it wasn't personal, but I didn't think she was going to tell the whole world. I don't really get rattled, though. To me, this wasn't that serious. If that's what she had to do to feel better, then that was what she had to do. It had a lot to do with her arguing with Dallas in the studio, and him critiquing the music she wanted to write and produce for TLC. I'd watch them argue and at one point it got ugly. It was a mess. She felt that he had too much power and it was her album. So if she couldn't work freely on the TLC album, she'd do her own. I did however demo every song she wrote for TLC but they still got turned down by the label.

And the truth is, I never had a problem with Lisa going solo. I did have an issue with when and how she decided to do it. She went about it all in the wrong way. TLC was in the middle of a contract with our record label, and we needed to finish and promote *FanMail*, but Lisa wanted to ditch us in the midst of it all to make a rap record with Suge Knight. It wasn't the right time. She had to finish what she started. I was annoyed because she kept skipping out on obligations and she thought her songs with Suge were more important than the commitment she made beforehand with TLC. She'd gone to California to record with him when she was supposed to be with us, and I let her have it. We'd booked studio time and she wasn't there.

"This is wack," I told Lisa over the phone. "Your music isn't even good yet. You don't have any hits." I was angry, so I was trying to hurt her because I felt disrespected, but it was true. I probably shouldn't have said it that way even if it was how I felt. I could have handled it better. But she was giving all this attitude and I wasn't lying. The music she was making with Suge could have been better. She was furious. She slammed down the phone and went straight to Suge. He retaliated for her. He asked people to dis me and Chilli on the radio, and he got Wendy Williams to insult me on a TV interview. It got so bad that D'mon asked Suge to have a sit-down meeting to squash the drama. Lisa refused to talk to me.

One of the worst fights TLC ever had came the week *FanMail* was released. We were in New York, staying at the Trump International Hotel & Tower. It's fancy and everything was coated in a lacquer of gold. Celebs had condos on the other side, too. We'd run into people like Steven Tyler and John Travolta there. I loved John in *Grease*, and I always did his dance in "Greased Lightning." Once I remember his son Jett jumping into my limo by mistake and I was so excited. The hotel was cool because people didn't think about Donald Trump the same way back then. Sleeping in one of his hotels equated to fame. We came in from Atlanta to appear on MTV's *Total Request Live* to promote the album, but Lisa was acting nuts thanks to her boyfriend she called Papi.

All that posh luxury was the opposite of our vibe at the time. There was so much strife between us, and it just kept growing. Lisa was never there when she was supposed to be, and we had this new record to sell. It started getting real. It was disrespectful not just to TLC but to everyone around us, especially people hired for events she didn't show up to, which always cost us money. Anyone who knows me knows that disrespect and I don't get along, but I'd remained calm, somehow, until now. I kept giving Lisa passes I wouldn't give to others. But this time I couldn't let it all slide.

The tension was high. Lisa was mostly avoiding me and Chilli. She spent all her time with Papi, who was a real piece of work. He tried to control everything she did. He was a married man who met Lisa when he brought his wife to audition for her, which I didn't know until his wife rang me up. I got this call while we were staying at the Trump Hotel and a woman said, "I'm looking for this bitch Lisa."

"Hold up," I said. "What?"

"This is Papi's wife," she said.

"Okay," I replied. "Back up. First, I don't mind helping you deliver whatever message you want to give your husband. But kick back with the cusswords. And I don't control grown people and their decisions. I didn't even know you existed until now."

"Tell my husband to call home," she told me, mentioning their kids. Great. So Papi had a wife and kids, and here he was on tour with TLC. Who knows—he could have lied to Lisa and said that he was no longer married. I had a lot of issues with Papi already. It seemed like he'd brainwashed Lisa. He was always in her ear, and she brought him to our band meetings. He once fired our sound guy. And she let him. Excuse me? This is TLC, not TLC and boyfriends. He didn't belong in these situations. So I never cared for him. During one particular argument, I hurled a Coke bottle at his head. I missed, but the fact was that I wanted to fight him. He was seriously taking advantage of Lisa. Watching it made my stomach turn. Love can be blind and the ones on the outside of the relationship can see more clearly.

After his wife hung up, I went straight out and said, in front of everybody, "Your wife said to call home." Lisa gave me a mean look. I didn't care. But he should know that his wife was calling up members of TLC and acting crazy. Of course, he kept sticking his nose in everything. That didn't stop him.

On the day of the *TRL* taping, Lisa waited until 30 minutes before we had to go live and asked us to come up to our manager Bill's hotel room. She was shouting her head off. "I don't know where the money at," she hollered at us. Her eyes were wild. Papi wasn't with her, but I knew he was somewhere nearby and he had coached her into saying this. He was always involved in whatever Lisa had to say, or they would come up with schemes together.

"I wanna know where the motherfucking money's at," Lisa yelled. "Puffy knows where the money's at. Master P knows where the money's at."

What money? At that time, Lisa had burned most of our bridges when she set fire to Andre's house. There was only one promoter left who wanted to take us on tour. No other promoter would touch us. Nike and Adidas didn't want us to wear their clothes anymore. The fans had started to sense our unrest. Not only were we not financially solid, but we were going to have to pay back any money advanced for our tour.

"I'm gonna get on live TV and tell everyone I'm not going on tour," Lisa said, her voice echoing off the walls. It was only Bill, Chilli, and me in the room. Everyone else was waiting in the lobby; the clock was ticking. We had minutes until we needed to appear on live TV.

"I'm not supporting it," she spat. "If motherfuckers weren't scared of doing what I was doing, then motherfuckers would be in a better position."

By motherfuckers she meant us, but she wasn't saying it directly. Chilli was over it, right away. She just stood up and walked out, the door smacking closed behind her. But I could feel myself getting worked up, the anger coming in fast. My face heated. Not only was I promoting TLC's new album, but I also had my own book *Thoughts* to worry about. If she ruined our tour, that would also ruin my chances of promoting my book and the book tour I had set up around TLC's tour schedule. It would mess up my chances of earning a solo living. I was ready to go do my own book tour if she refused to hit the road with TLC. But it couldn't be the way she wanted to do it. Did she really think I was about to let her walk out of this hotel, go live on TV, and embarrass us on *TRL*? She was the one who got us in this situation in the first place.

Bill tried to explain TLC's state of affairs the best he could. I got really quiet, which is never a good sign. Bill was worried about the time and told us we had to leave for the taping. He herded us out of the room and summoned Chilli to meet us downstairs. I met up with Nechole in the hallway, where she was waiting for me. Lisa's words were ringing in my ears as we all walked to the elevators. Lisa kept fussing and saying, "Motherfuckers should have done this or that," over and over, but never actually saying who she was talking about. The doors of the elevator closed. The walls were solid gold and shiny bright. I stared at my reflection, trying to channel my rage. But I was tired of Lisa's talk, tired of her boyfriend—all of it. As the elevator began to descend, I detonated.

"Say who the fuck the motherfucker is," I told Lisa, my finger extending toward her. I tapped her forehead. She didn't flinch. "Who you calling a motherfucker? Call me a motherfucker and I'm going to fuck you up."

We spilled out of the elevator into the hotel lobby and I continued to shout, "Call me a motherfucker. I dare you! I'm gonna beat your ass." I knew I couldn't actually beat her up since that wouldn't change things, but I wanted to.

She yelled back at me, still trying to argue her point about the money. She wouldn't acknowledge that I was about to hit her right there in the lobby of the Trump Hotel. Everybody was looking at us. I followed right behind her, yelling, "Say who! Say it!" Nechole tried to grab my finger, and I yelled, "Don't touch me."

Lisa ran down the front steps and found Papi, who was waiting for her. She stood beside him and gave me a look. "Now?" she said. Like that was going to stop anything. He didn't know that both me and Nechole were prepared to fight him, too.

"What's wrong?" Papi said. "What happened?"

"You know what happened," I retorted. "You sent this bitch to come tell me this bullshit. I'll tell you this—neither one of you is coming to *TRL*. Come down there and it will be the best show they ever had because I'm going to whip your ass on live TV."

I leaned back to Lisa. "If you gonna say something on live TV, then I'm going to make it a great show," I added.

Lisa walked toward the limo, yelling back.

"If you get in that car, on my life, I will whoop your ass," I promised her. The street was crowded with people and cars. She got in the car waiting to take us to the MTV studio. I banged on the window. My fist left a print on the glass.

"Don't come down there," I said again.

Lisa emerged as quickly as she'd gotten in, now crying. Without a word, she went back into the hotel, Papi trailing behind, probably plotting his next idiotic move. Didn't he know he was making this situation worse? He didn't care because he had an agenda.

Chilli and I went to *TRL* alone. Once the cameras started to roll, we smiled pretty. We were good at pretending to be carefree and fun because that's what we did all the time. And anyway, I'd won—for the time being.

"Obviously we're one short," *TRL* host Carson Daly told the studio audience. There was a crowd of people on the Times Square street outside MTV, waving signs with our name on it and yelling. They didn't know we were imploding. "We're missing the L in TLC, Left Eye," Carson said. "Is she okay?"

"Well," Chilli said, fidgeting, "don't get mad, but she don't feel good."

"She doesn't feel good," I affirmed.

"Is it a flu thing?" Carson asked. He didn't seem to know what to do. "Is it the upper respiratory thing that seems to be going around?"

"Well, we all got here last night," Chilli told him. "And all I have to say is Imodium A-D put it together." She quickly turned away from the cameras to hide her grin while I laughed gleefully into the microphone.

"I can't believe you just said that," Carson said, looking bewildered. "Left Eye is throwing stuff at the TV right now if she's watching."

After we got off the air, my mama called me.

"You hit Lisa," she accused me.

"I didn't hit Lisa," I retorted. "I said I was gonna hit her. There's a big difference."

Fans found out about that fight later. TLC went to do a photo shoot for *Entertainment Weekly*, and by then Chilli and I'd had it. Lisa left early to have a meeting with Puffy. She just left midway through, no concern for the photographer, the reporter, the makeup artist, the stylist, or us. We'd booked and paid for an entire crew of people and rented the studio where the shoot was taking place. After she disappeared, we let loose, even though the public had already noticed what was going on. We admitted that Lisa was undermining the promotion of our album, that she'd been ditching rehearsals, that she constantly threatened to quit, which had caused some problems with LaFace. We were so tired of it. But we also couldn't hide it because she left in front of the reporter. The reporter asked and we told the truth. We revealed that Lisa hadn't been sick during *TRL*. After the interview, *Entertainment Weekly* ran a story in October of 1999, months after the album had dropped, called "Are TLC about to Sing the Breakup Blues?" Our talking only seemed to make Lisa act worse. She tried to cover up her behavior when they called her for a comment after our interview, but a few weeks later, the magazine ran a follow-up article.

"I challenge Tionne 'Player' Watkins and Rozonda 'Hater' Thomas to an album entitled *The Challenge*," Lisa wrote in a statement she sent in. "A 3 CD set that contains three solo albums. I also challenge Dallas 'The Manipulator' Austin to produce all of the material and do it at a fraction of his normal rate. As I think about it, I'm sure LaFace would not mind throwing in a 1.5 million dollar prize for the winner. *Billboard* will determine the winner."

"I just want to present the challenge—they don't have to take it," Lisa explained to the magazine. "I just want credit for my ideas, because I am the creative force behind TLC." Ummm . . . no. Maybe one of the creative forces but not the only. Do you know how many things I've done in TLC that I didn't take credit for? I was raised not to brag or play the "me, me, me" game. If I did something, it would come to light when needed and people would find out by word of mouth. I was thinking, did she forget all the things we did together, just her and me? For example, how she had come up with the album title and I had come up with the album cover and what we were wearing. Afterward she told me that it wasn't me she was mad at or gunning for. It was others around us, such as certain producers or label heads who didn't give her credit. Later I found that to be true on many occasions when it started to happen to me.

This statement wasn't what TLC was about, anyway. I wasn't down. We were a group, and everything we'd made had been done together. Unity was needed, not division. It stung. And it pissed me off because she was calling us names and saw things differently than I did, some of it accurate and some of it not so much. Chilli and I weren't about to take Lisa up on this. We released our own statement in response.

"Unity does not mean we will all believe in or do the same things," we wrote. "It means we will agree to do something without battling over how and why."

Papi stuck around for a while after the *TRL* incident, even though we all knew he had a family back home. He helped Lisa write all these letters and statements to the press. She acted weirder and weirder as the time went on. She wasn't herself. If I said, "What's wrong with you?" she would just reply, "Nothing." At one interview, I said hi and she greeted me like a stranger. I couldn't imagine what Papi was saying to her behind closed doors. I knew she was upset with me because I didn't agree with her.

I didn't hold a grudge, and things cooled down some as we toured on *FanMail*, but I didn't spend a lot of time with Lisa anymore. At one point, she and I were inseparable. It wasn't like our early tours. We weren't running through any hallways or getting into trouble. Chilli and I got the message that we shouldn't talk to Lisa—or even touch her. Of course, that wasn't going to fly with me. I went out onstage one night and wrapped my arms around her. She barely reacted. I loved her even if she was mad.

The communication was minimal as we played show after show. Lisa had an assistant named Tab, and she would send Tab to bring me letters about anything that was amiss. If Lisa was unhappy with management, it would show up in a letter. I wanted to talk to her, but she wouldn't engage. There were no conversations, even though she was sitting next to me half the time. One day Tab brought me another letter.

"If you come in here with one more letter, I'm gonna beat your ass," I said.

"But, Tionne, I don't have nothing to do with it," Tab said.

"Yes you do," I replied. "You're the one bringing the letters. So now you're in it. Tell her if you bring me any more letters I'm gonna beat your ass."

Tab didn't bring me any more letters. Lisa loosened up a little bit. I think it was because I wouldn't buy into her nonsense. She started coming back around, and we would talk sometimes. We didn't party anymore, though, and it wasn't the same. We played the songs and gave whatever we could to our fans. There was no more talk of breaking up. The drama may have even helped, in some ways. *FanMail* went to No. 1 on the *Billboard* 200, and we were nominated for eight more Grammys, including for Album of the Year.

TLC continued, but Lisa remained somewhat distant. We all had our own lives and started doing more things outside of TLC. Later, after we'd finished touring on *FanMail*, she pretended to go missing. She skipped out on a press conference we had scheduled in Las Vegas at the end of August, and the newspapers reported that people around her were worried. Everyone speculated. Did she run off? Was she abducted? The fans freaked out. But Lisa pulled things like this. She thought it was funny. And she loved the press. She and her new boyfriend Sean Newman were actually bouncing around the country, and we knew she was fine. The press ate it up. Where was Lisa? Had someone really spotted her in New Orleans? I didn't want to play along.

At that time, I was pregnant with Chase. Lisa and I were mostly on the outs. We were living our own lives, but enough was enough. I called her up.

"Stop it," I told her. "A lot of people have loved ones who go missing for real. This isn't funny." Being pregnant made me feel even more sensitive about it.

She didn't like that, but I couldn't stand what she was doing. It wasn't a joke.

"Whatever," she replied. But she emerged. She showed up with us to the MOBO Awards in London, which honored black artists, in October. Lisa tried to claim that her disappearance was for publicity. "All publicity is good publicity," she said. But that isn't always true. There's publicity and then there's selfish antics. After that, the public didn't hear much from us or from Lisa. It was best to just live our lives and think about the next album, which we were starting to make.

In 2001, TLC was invited to perform at MTV's 20th anniversary party, MTV20: Live and Almost Legal, at the Hammerstein Ballroom in New York. It was a ton of artists: Mary J. Blige, Mariah Carey, Billy Idol. We played "Waterfalls," and it was kind of strange to be back onstage with TLC after all the strife. I put everything aside. If you love someone you move forward. I had said my piece and moved on, hoping that TLC would put this behind us and become even stronger. But we didn't realize it would be our final performance together. That night, onstage in New York, was the last time Lisa, Chilli, and I played as one.

CHAPTER 8

BC/AC

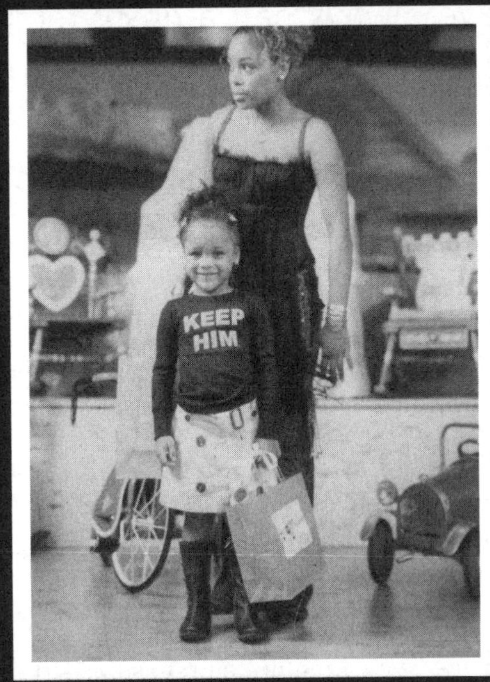

My life has had two eras: BC and AC. They are divided by the birth of my daughter, Chase, who changed everything for me. Before she arrived, I was a very different sort of person. I've always had a quick temper. If someone comes at me, it won't turn out well. Same thing with a 6-foot man. I should run or be afraid, but I'm not, and that's the problem.

I've come home with black eyes or with blood dripping down my head. I've had to say, "Wash this out; it ain't my blood." I've fought in the street. When things weren't working exactly like I wanted them to, I got pissed. I was a time bomb, continuously ticking. My mama always said, "Tionne, your temper's so bad. You can die like that!"

There are a few infamous stories about my temper, all incidents that happened during the BC era. In recent years, I've heard people use the phrase "Don't make me T-Boz you," which is apparently now slang for a physical threat. But it's true—I've gotten myself into some situations.

My worst moment of rage came in 1996, at the height of

TLC's early fame. To this day, my mama believes that I broke my hand because it was slammed in a car door. But that's not the real truth.

Dalvin, who was my boyfriend at the time, was visiting Charlotte, North Carolina, where he was from. He was staying in a hotel and had an adjoining room with this girl Kim, whom he called his cousin. She wasn't actually his cousin—she was a recording artist he'd known for a long time and he'd worked with. That night, way past midnight, he got drunk and fell asleep while we were on the phone. I was trying to get him to wake up and go take a shower. Evidently, he had way too much to drink, and I didn't know what that was like since I don't drink.

"Dalvin," I said firmly, "get up."

Nothing. I tried this for almost 15 minutes. But he wouldn't wake up. He just kept sleeping with the phone apparently still in his hand.

"No, no, no." I suddenly heard Kim's voice in the background. She sounded stressed out. "You can't come in here," she was saying. "What are you doing?"

There was a moment of silence and some shuffling and someone else picked up the phone.

"Hello?" It was a girl's voice. "Who's this?"

"Angel," I lied. "Who's this?"

"Mimi," she said. Ah, shit. It was that bitch he used to go with when he was younger. (For the record, Mimi is not her real name. But let's call her that for the sake of the story.) She was always trying to get back with him and always talking crap about me. I put up with her talking trash for years and always turned the other cheek, but this time I'd had enough. Here was an opportunity and I was taking it.

"Why are you there?" I asked.

"I'm 'bout to get my man back," she replied.

"Don't he have a girlfriend?" I said. "That girl in TLC?"

"Yeah," she said. "So?"

Nope. That pissed me off. "Okay, bitch," I replied. "I'll see you in a minute."

I hung up, threw on a T-shirt, some sweatpants, and sneakers. I grabbed a Taser, this pen that could be transformed into a knife, $5,000 in cash for bail, and left my house at 5:00 a.m. I got on the first flight out of Atlanta an hour later. It was only 45 minutes on the plane from Atlanta to Charlotte, and I was fuming the whole way. I was so tired of this girl. She needed to know who she was fucking with. I was taking this special flight just to beat her ass.

I took a cab to the hotel. "Hi," I said to the clerk at the front desk. "I'd like to pay for an extra night for room 420. I'll need another key, please." He took my cash and handed me the key. I stomped up to the room, ready to throw down.

I slid the key into the door and threw it open. Kim looked up, instantly concerned. My boyfriend was still passed out from the night before, laying across his bed in his pants and socks but no shirt, and that bitch Mimi was in the bed with him, just lying there. She saw me.

"Oh, shit," she said.

"Yeah, bitch," I replied. I yanked back the covers on the bed. She had on a T-shirt and no panties. That set me off. And I wasn't just mad at her. It was his fault, too. In my head, they'd already had sex. Or he'd at least let her in the bed. And now I had to deal with her. I was at the highest point of pissed off that a human could be.

I grabbed Mimi's leg and dragged her off the bed with only one hand. She smacked onto the floor and I fell on top of her, not realizing how strong I was. I wrapped her hair around my hand several times until she couldn't move her head. Then I went to work on her face, slamming my fist into her eye over and over. As I was punching her, Dalvin finally woke up.

"What the hell is going on?" he said. He yelled for Kim to come help.

"Don't move," I said, still whaling on her face. "I'll fuck you up. Don't touch me. Nobody moves."

Mimi's face turned black and blue, and I could feel the crunch of her cheekbone under my fist—or maybe it was the bones in my own hand; I couldn't tell. But that didn't stop me. Dalvin finally got up and tried to pull me off, asking Kim to grab me.

"No," I said, pointing at Kim. I was still holding the girl's hair with my other hand. I waggled my finger at her. "I'll fuck you up, too. I swear to God," I added. She stopped in her tracks for a minute. But somehow they tackled me off her, despite my threats. Mimi jumped up and ran.

"This is your fault," I spat at Dalvin. I swung at him, and then I shoved him off me and ran after her. She had a head start. All the maids were staring at me as I hurtled past them. "Isn't that the girl from TLC?" I heard one of them say.

"Where'd she go?" I shouted.

"That way," one of the maids told me, gesturing down the stairs. But Mimi was gone. I went back to the hotel room, ready to fuck him up, too. I leapt at him, going in for the jugular.

"I didn't know," he insisted. "I swear! I was knocked out." Who cared? He had to be responsible for his own stupid actions. I climbed off him and sat down. My hand started tingling and burning, the pain coming in. As I was sitting there, rubbing my swollen fingers, the phone rang. It was her. She clearly was crazy.

"Put her on speaker," I said. He clicked the button. "What is your problem?" I asked her. "You just got your ass kicked and you're calling back here."

"I had him first," she said, sounding pathetic. "Then you came along."

"How could I take him when you dated when you were teenagers?" I said. "Do you want me to fuck you up again? What is your issue? Do you know how many chicks he's been with since you? If I find you, I'm gonna finish what I started." She hung up. I just wanted to go home.

"I don't care if you knew or not," I told Dalvin as the phone clicked off. "It's your fault she exists. She's part of your crazy package."

I couldn't get a flight home that day, so Dalvin's mom got us another hotel room. I didn't want to go to the hospital, even though my hand started throbbing and swelling up. The adrenaline was wearing off. I didn't want to talk to anyone. Dalvin stayed with me, trying to get me back in his good graces all night. But I didn't care. A ton of emotions ran through me. I was mad, hurt, disgusted, and just plain sad. I got on a flight first thing the next day and went straight from the airport to the emergency room. My hand was broken.

Later that day, my hand in a cast, my phone rang. It was my lawyer.

"I got the funniest call," he said. "I think someone mixed up the band members—this has to be Left Eye that they're talking about. There's this girl who is so fucked up. Her eye socket is broken, her jaw is cracked, and her whole left side of her face is bruised. They said you came in her room and beat her up." I got really quiet, then explained.

"Well, technically, I paid to get into that room," I said. "And it wasn't her room. I went into my boyfriend's room with a key I paid for." Obviously, the hotel wasn't supposed to do that. "And it was me," I confirmed. "Not Lisa."

He literally dropped the phone in disbelief. I could hear him scrambling to pick it back up. "I can't believe you did this," he said when he'd recovered.

"Well, I did," I replied. "And my mom doesn't know, so we're going to keep this between us. She thinks I spent the night at a friend's and I broke my hand slamming it into a car door. So let's figure this out."

We got Mimi to drop the lawsuit. I called her not knowing she was still in the hospital (years later I found out she had to stay there for 2 months to let her face heal). "It would be in your best interest to drop this," I said. "If you don't, I'm gonna pick up your face where I left off." And so it went away. I never felt bad about beating her up, but it did make me reconsider my temper. I knew my rage was something I needed to fix. I never planned to hurt her so badly, but it happened.

I got in so many fights back then, although none quite as bad as that one. And from my perspective, I never started them. I was just reacting to anybody who messed with me. Another infamous story took place shortly before Chase was born, when I'd gotten out of the hospital from a sickle cell crisis. I stopped by my favorite restaurant on my way home. As I was sitting at the counter with my security guard Dave and my cousin Marde, I noticed two elderly black women standing at the register for a while waiting to pay. The waitress was ignoring them. She was wasting time, not doing her job at all, and it bothered me.

"Excuse me," I said loudly. "They need help." I gestured toward the two women. The waitress looked at me and walked over to cash them out. Then she came over to my seat.

"Can I take your order?" She said it with such an attitude. I wanted to let it go and turn the other cheek. "Okay," I thought to myself, "you're just cranky because you're coming off your hospital meds." I took a deep breath.

"The southwestern pasta with extra blackened shrimp," I said, as politely as I could manage. It was the same order I got there two or three times a week. It was supposed to come with six shrimp, but I always ordered extra and I always asked for extra sauce. When we came in, they called us the "extra family" because everything we ordered involved something additional.

When the waitress came back with my food, there were only three shrimp on the plate. So not only did she ignore the fact that I asked for extra, she brought me less than it was supposed to come with.

"Excuse me," I said, calling her over. She took her sweet time coming. "This is supposed to have six shrimp," I said. "And I paid for extra. And I asked for extra sauce."

She glared at me and walked away. When she came back, she had a big-ass cup in her hand. She smacked it down on the counter in front of me. Bam! But there was barely any sauce in it. Not to mention that Dave and Marde were still waiting for their food. I couldn't figure out what her issue was. But after a few minutes, I realized it: She was hurrying to help all of the white customers in the restaurant. It was just the black customers who didn't seem to deserve her attention.

"Excuse me," I said again. I wanted my extra shrimp and

my sauce. But I also wanted to make a point. She couldn't pick and choose which customers to help based on the color of their skin. There was no response. "Excuse me!" I yelled it this time.

She stepped out. "What? I am trying to fix your order," she screamed back.

"Who the fuck are you talking to?" I replied. My temper was rising up.

"You!" she yelled. I swear I heard her mutter the n-word under her breath.

My face flushed. Thirty minutes had gone by since we arrived. I was just trying to get some pasta on my way out of a painful hospital visit, and I hit my boiling point. I took the cup of sauce she slammed down on the counter and hurled it at her. It spread across the counter, onto her and across Dave's bald head and neck. I didn't notice right away that it had burned him. He was fine—no scarring—and laughed it off, but I still felt bad.

The waitress was shocked and ready to come at me, but I was way ahead of her. I stood up on my chair and tried to jump over the bar. My cousin grabbed me. She'd seen me do this before at a Dairy Queen when the girl got my order wrong and had snatched it out of my hand to replace it, scratching me in the process. I jumped over the counter and popped that girl in the face and was banned from that Dairy Queen, so Marde knew when to hold me back. Marde knew I was always ready to fight and that my temper was endless when I felt provoked.

"Time to go," my cousin said, pulling me away. We left before the cops could show, and I threw that shrimp pasta in the trash on my way out. There was no telling what she did to it.

But that felt normal for me, fighting and yelling and standing up for myself when I was wronged. My temper had been like that for as long as I could remember. Things were like that before Chase was born. I didn't care who I hurt or threatened or what it cost me. I never started the fights, in my opinion, but I always joined them. And since I had no one to worry about but myself, I didn't ever think anything was wrong with this. But in 2000, everything changed. Chase was a true miracle. The doctors had said I could never get pregnant because of my sickle cell, and I'd also had a fibroid cyst removed from my uterus. Chase made me into a new person.

It all began at the 42nd Annual Grammys, although I didn't realize it at the time. I've never liked going to awards shows—unless I'm performing, working, or winning. Most are boring as all get-out. I'd sit in that crowd for hours and just want to choke myself unless good artists were playing. The best ones were when Prince or Michael Jackson played, but neither of them were on deck for the Grammys that year. It was February of 2000, right after we'd headlined the FanMail Tour with Destiny's Child and Christina Aguilera opening for us. We were nominated for eight awards, all for *FanMail*, and that was the only reason I wanted to go. Plus, if the Grammys ask you to perform, you do it if you're smart.

You probably remember those Grammys for the green Versace dress Jennifer Lopez wore. The one with the jungle print and the really low-cut neck. It had a slit from her throat all the way down to her coochie. I'll never forget how much attention she got when she walked the red carpet, all the photographers screaming for a good shot. I remember thinking, "That's a bad-ass dress." I remembered seeing it on the runway. Man, she wore that dress hunty.

TLC usually got "Best Dressed" after awards shows (even when we had to compete with J-Lo and all her good stuff), but this year I was pissed because I had a wardrobe malfunction. You can't see it in the photos, but I almost had a booby slip while we performed. I wore a black jacket and black thigh-high stockings that looked like pants, which was a quick fix from the original ensemble. The main issue was that my boobs were perking right out of it, changing the look of the outfit. I'd always been a member of the itty-bitty-titty committee, but for some reason they'd popped up in the last month and they were sore. It was something I noticed, but didn't really think much about it. I figured, "Maybe boobs just start to grow at some point."

J-Lo, her dress, and David Duchovny announced our win for Best R&B Album, which set the evening off right. Over the course of the night—which was so long—we took home three of the eight awards we'd been up for. It was exciting. Even if awards bored me sometimes, I loved to win, and I appreciate the fans for making it all possible (although I'm always nervous to give our acceptance speeches). But in all of the photos of us on the red carpet, in the video of us performing, what I didn't realize was that I had a passenger along for the ride.

After the Grammys we were supposed to spend 2 extra days in LA shooting a video for the Goodie Mob's new single "What It Ain't." TLC was the featured artist on the song, and the video treatment involved me and Lisa and Chilli hanging out in a diner and then dancing around a warehouse club. It was us and the Goodie Mob versus some aliens. The director, David Meyers, wanted something edgy and fun, and the shoot was planned for Johnie's Broiler in Downey, a restaurant famous for its '50s vibe (and for appearing in a bunch of movies). But when we arrived on set, something was off.

I felt really weird. I was dizzy and my booby cakes, now gigantic (for me, anyway), ached. In my trailer, I lay down and rubbed my chest. I was used to my body acting up—you go to work, maybe you feel like shit, and then you do the work anyway—but this wasn't right. And the weirdest thing wasn't the pain or the wooziness. It was that I wanted a Subway sandwich.

The truth is, I didn't care for Subway as much as Blimpie. I've always liked Blimpie better. I order the Blimpie Best with provolone cheese, extra onions, and no tomatoes on white bread, and it's my favorite. So why would I want a Spicy Italian sub from Subway? It didn't make any sense.

"I think you're pregnant," my assistant and friend Nechole joked, sitting with me in the trailer.

"I can't have babies," I retorted, certain. I was aching all over. I didn't feel right. I went to the director and apologized.

"I don't think I can do this video today," I said. I hated having to admit that I wasn't feeling well. I worried that people thought I was always messing things up. I wanted to work through the pain. The director looked me up and down.

"You need to go to the hospital," he said. "We can pick up your scenes later."

Nechole took me into the hospital and called D'mon to meet us there. I assumed this was just another flare-up of sickle cell, which is called a sickle cell crisis. Maybe I was overworked.

The emergency room doctor came in and asked me what was wrong. "I feel super weird," I said. "And I want Subway and I don't even really like Subway."

The doctor suggested an x-ray, just to check what was going on. But Nechole stopped him.

"She needs a urinalysis test," Nechole said. She had worked for years at a medical clinic. "I think she's pregnant. No x-rays until we're sure."

"I can't have babies," I said, again. "Come on, Nechole."

"We'll be thorough," the doctor assured us. "We'll check everything."

"Okay," I said. "Whatever." Better safe than sorry, but I still thought it was a waste of time.

The ER doctor told the nurse, "Test her for pregnancy. She's been craving sandwiches." The nurse took some blood from my arm and ran me through some tests, then vanished.

I waited in the ER room with Nechole and D'mon, believing none of it. There was no way I was pregnant.

But a little while later the ER doctor returned, armed with some papers. "So," he said, "do you want everyone to stay in the room while I give you your results?" I nodded. No one moved. "Well," he said. "You *are* pregnant."

"Nope," I replied. Was this guy serious? I'd been told my whole life that babies were impossible. Was this a joke? I thought I was being punked and Ashton Kutcher was going to jump out any second. The doctor had to be wrong.

D'mon grinned. "You're pregnant!" he said. Nechole started jumping around the room, gleeful. She looked so pleased with herself for knowing.

I dialed my mama. "Mama," I said, "I'm pregnant." There was a long pause. Maybe she hadn't heard me. "Oh, Lordy Jesus," she said. "Oh, Lordy Jesus." She said it three times, louder every time. "Oh, Lordy Jesus." Nothing else came out. I couldn't tell if she was mad or excited.

"We're going to admit you for a few days," the doctor said. "We just want to monitor things and get your sickle cell crisis under control." But as I lay there, I couldn't come to terms with the news. It seemed impossible. I was afraid to be happy in case the doctor was wrong. After endless questions and skepticism from me, they finally sent me upstairs to admit me into a hospital room.

That's where I met Dr. Raymond Poliakin for the first time a few days later. He had a bunch of paperwork with him. "So you don't believe you're really pregnant," he said, smiling.

"Nope," I said.

"I am very confident that you *are* pregnant," Dr. Poliakin affirmed.

But my mind was still scrambling to make sense of those words. "Test me again and then show me the numbers," I told him. "I just don't believe it. I've been told my whole life that I can't have babies. Are you sure you didn't get my test results mixed up with some other lady?"

Dr. Poliakin waited for me to catch my breath and then handed me a piece of paper. "Here are the numbers," he said, pointing. "Honey, you are very, *very* pregnant."

The truth. I was pregnant. Very, *very* pregnant. His words kept repeating in my head. I was convinced they'd messed up, the way the doctors were always messing up. What if they came back and told me it was a mistake? What if the test was wrong? What if it didn't stick? But underneath, under the disbelief, I could feel a surge of happiness. I was going to have a baby.

The news changed everything I thought I knew about myself. I'd been told the same thing for so many years by so many doctors, and I'd believed it. I'd imagined a different possibility, of course, talking to D'mon about having a kid. Hoping for a miracle. But if you're told something over and over, you eventually start to believe it's real. Sometimes, in the back of your mind, your brain won't stop questioning it, but when everyone keeps saying things, it starts to mess with your mind. No babies for me. I kept thinking, "Is this really happening?" But it was.

So now I had to reassess what was true. I already knew doctors could get it wrong. They're wrong all the fucking time. But could they get it this wrong? I know miracles happen, but could I be experiencing one for myself? Maybe God really did have a plan.

My mama didn't want me to get my hopes up too high, especially when the pregnancy was still new. "Don't jinx it," she said. "Wait until after your fourth or fifth month. Some people miscarry or the pregnancy doesn't stick. Don't go buying any baby clothes yet." So instead I'd go to the mall and look at the clothes in the stores. We didn't know if it was a boy or a girl, but I'd run my fingers over the tiny little shoes and miniature dresses, imagining which ones I'd get.

Four months passed and the chances of miscarriage decreased almost to zero. The baby was holding on tight. I started to buy baby clothes, stockpiling them for later. People sent me gifts and those piled up, too. When we found out I was pregnant, D'mon was living in a mansion in Calabasas and I had a house in Atlanta. We used to fly back and forth, because I didn't believe in shacking up before marriage, but once we knew this baby was coming, we bought a townhouse in Westlake Village. Before that, we had been living in the Beverly Hills Hotel for some months, paying cash for the room.

Pregnancy was hard. I felt so tired as the baby settled inside me, and my disease flared up every once in a while. While we were looking for houses, D'mon and our Realtor would often find me lying down in one of the rooms, exhausted. I couldn't take my usual pain medications while hospitalized for any sickle cell crisis because the doctors didn't want the baby to get addicted to the high-powered drugs that help keep my pain under control. So I had to suffer through. Whatever they gave me didn't work or wasn't strong enough. It really hurt sometimes. Some days my joints ached and there was nothing I could do about it.

It's strange being inside a body that feels like it stops being entirely your own. My boobs continued to blow up, going from a 34B to a 36DDD. I gained only 18 pounds overall, but it was all BBBB: baby, booty, boobies, and belly. Everything, by all accounts I'd heard, was normal. But I was nervous. I couldn't stop worrying that something would go wrong. I went to the doctor twice a week. Sometimes three times.

"Just check," I'd say. "Make sure the baby isn't all twisted in the umbilical cord." A few days later: "Check me again."

I was there so often that I made friends with the nurses and the doctor. We'd eat lunch together. The doctor even invited me over to his house to get to know his family. I was probably such a pest, but they didn't seem to mind. Every time I showed up at the office, one of the nurses would say, "It's okay, honey," and show me straight back.

I kept working throughout the pregnancy, and it wasn't a secret from my fans that I was preggo. I made two music videos with D'mon, one for our single "Tight to Def." At the beginning of the video, which is a modern-day *Bonnie and*

Clyde story, you can see him rubbing my growing belly as I'm standing next to a car in a tight black dress. Later, I made a video for "My Getaway," the title track for the animated film *Rugrats in Paris*. Somehow you can't even tell I'm pregnant in that video. Although now, when I look back, I can tell in my face that something was different.

Midway through the pregnancy, on August 19, D'mon and I got married by the ocean at the Trump National Golf Club in Palos Verdes. It was massive and elaborate, and there were 10 bridesmaids, 10 groomsmen, and nearly 300 guests. The colors were natural tones, with everyone in white and tan. It was one of the most beautiful weddings I've ever seen—and I'm not just saying that because it was my own. My husband's favorite group, The Whispers, played the reception, and the late, great Gerald Levert sang me down the aisle. Chilli was there, but Lisa wasn't. She didn't come, which has always made me sad.

I had a lot of conflicted feelings that day, not because Lisa skipped out, but because my hormones were revving high. Planning the wedding had been exhausting. Even as I was smiling, I kept thinking, "Am I making a mistake? Do you think he's cheating on me?" Those thoughts got worse during the bachelor party the night before the wedding because, well, you know what most men do.

It was a lot to manage. My dress was too heavy for me, but very beautiful. It was ivory with a long embroidered train design by Monique Lhuillier and was worth $48,000. I got it for free if I featured it in *INStyle* magazine. I was completely wiped out by the time the reception ended. My body went into a sickle cell crisis, and we had to cancel our honeymoon so I could go to the hospital. I lay in bed, pain running through my body, instead of celebrating the way a husband and wife are meant to celebrate. It was a beautiful wedding, but if I had to do it again, I would never have something so big and involved. It was beyond stressful.

After the wedding, D'mon and I bought a house in Camarillo on 5 acres of land to replace the townhouse. I decorated the nursery and finally believed it was all happening. Now, I just had to wait for the baby to arrive.

I didn't have to wait long, as it turned out. On October 20, 2000, my daughter Chase Anela Rolison was born, arriving 1 month and 4 days early. I had a C-section, purposefully. Chilli was supposed to throw me a baby shower. We'd planned for everyone to come the weekend of my C-section appointment for a shower and slumber party. The idea was that everyone would spend the night and then come see my daughter born. But things didn't go that way, so I never got the shower.

I'd decided early on that I never wanted to push out a baby. My coochie was staying exactly how it was, thank you. No way I'd shove a person out of there. I didn't even want to deal with my water breaking. I'd seen her head on the ultrasound, and it was huge, just like her dad's, and there was no way I was thrusting that out of my body.

I stopped at Subway on my way to the hospital for a routine checkup, weeks before the scheduled C-section. I was still craving those sandwiches and I had to get one. When I got to the hospital, the baby wasn't moving. Dr. Poliakin hooked me up to some monitors while I was eating my spicy Italian sub, and suddenly all these nurses and hospital workers busted into the room. "We need to have the baby right now," someone said.

"Wait, what?" I wasn't ready. All these random people were

making me feel frantic. And I had a sandwich in my hand.

"Out," Dr. Poliakin told them, shooing them out the door. "Don't worry," he told me. "Your baby's heartbeat has slowed down, so it's time to get her out. We're going to take her out early." I didn't know they had 20 minutes to deliver Chase or she might not have survived.

I remember moments of the C-section, but not everything. It's blurry in places. I remember lying on the table with this blue sheet blocking the view of my lower half and a light above, glaring in my face. My arms had to stay flat across these boards, which was really uncomfortable.

"Are you sure I'm numb?" I asked, more than once.

"Can you feel this?" Dr. P replied. Nothing. "We're poking your toe with a very sharp object," he said. Still nothing. I didn't feel it when he cut into my belly.

But there was a complication: Chase was stuck under my rib cage because my torso is so short. She was all the way up at the top of my abs, above where the doctor was about to numb me.

"Okay," he told me in a calm voice. "We're going to push her down." He placed his hands under my ribs. "Take a deep breath." I inhaled and felt an insane pressure coming down on my chest. It hurt. A lot.

And then, suddenly, Chase was there. He lifted her over the blue sheet and I thought, "She's so pretty. She looks like my mom."

As I thought of my own mother, who had just left town thinking I wouldn't give birth yet, tears began to stream down my face. I was sorry for everything I had ever put her through, sorry for all the worry I'd caused. I felt instantly guilty for everything bad I'd ever done. I remembered all my fights, all the irrational moments of anger. "I hope my daughter doesn't do that to me," I thought. "I hope she's better than I was."

The first time I sat alone with Chase, after the doctor had stitched me up and the nurses had settled me into a hospital room, I was flooded with feelings. I lowered my face to her skin and wondered how anything could smell so pure and so fresh. She had this amazingly sweet smell, and she had pouty little lips and pale hair and green, charcoal, and hazel eyes, like swirled marble. She was perfect. I thought, "I can't believe I made this. I can't believe I made this little person and such a beautiful baby."

It's a very surreal experience to sit alone with a human being you created. It's weird when your own child, so small and new, stares into your eyes. It was like she knew me. She had my mama's eyes, and I felt like I was looking at my mom through her. She was what I'd been told I could never have, and now I had her. Ever since, whenever I've been asked, I've always said, "Chase is my greatest accomplishment."

I'd been holding on to the name Chase for a while. D'mon and I had talked about several names, including Chance, but Chase is the one that stuck. All these ideas for names came from liking my godsister's son's name. I'd even been calling myself Chase Rolison as an alias while out on the road with TLC. I told D'mon, "I'm going to call myself Chase until we have a baby," even before we knew it was possible we could have one. Her middle name, Anela, means "angel" in Hawaiian.

We had to stay in the hospital for 9 days after Chase was born because I was still having a crisis. On the first night, after Chase was born, the nurses told me I needed to breastfeed her. "The baby needs colostrum," they said. They kept repeating those sorts of phrases: "The baby needs this" and "The baby needs that." I didn't know any better, so I agreed. It seemed like the right thing to do. And they make you feel so guilty if you don't pop your titties out for the baby immediately. No bottle formula or you're a bad mother.

But sickle cell patients need every drop of fluid they can get, and losing that much breast milk shocked my body and almost stopped my heart. Every time Chase latched on, I would vomit and lose more fluids. But I felt forced to do it. Eventually, my body shut down and I fell into a coma. I spent 3 days unconscious in the ICU with my newborn daughter waiting for me to wake up.

When I did finally wake, everything was blurry. My eyelids felt heavy. My mama was there, along with several nurses. Chase wasn't in the room. "Go get her baby," my mama told one of the nurses. I could hear the urgency in her voice. "Go."

I blinked at the fluorescent lights. The room felt alien. Suddenly, the nurse was there holding Chase. She was so small, her fingers curled so tight. "Put the baby on her heart," my mama said. "Lay her down." And then Chase was stretched out over the left side of my chest, her heart beating against mine.

"Tionne," my mama said, "you have to fight. You have someone to live for."

Chase breathed slowly on top of me. I could feel her, alive, against me. She was definitely something to live for.

When I woke fully, once my mama was convinced I was not going to fall back into the coma, I held Chase in my arms. Her arrival was not just the beginning of her life, but of my own, too.

I decided that my life would be divided into two eras: "Before Chase" and "After Chase." I would try to change my life for the better. I would try to turn the other cheek when people made me angry. No more jumping over counters or putting my hands on people. I couldn't make any promises, but I wanted to try. From now on, whenever I wanted to whoop someone's ass, I'd say to myself, "She gets a Chase pass." And, for the record, I don't plan on breaking any more faces in the future.

All jokes aside, I had a daughter. Now, if I died, I'd leave someone behind. She was born against all odds, and she gave me something to live for. She changed everything. All the days before Chase were BC, and all those after were AC.

CHAPTER 9

RIP LeLe, Lisa, Left Eye

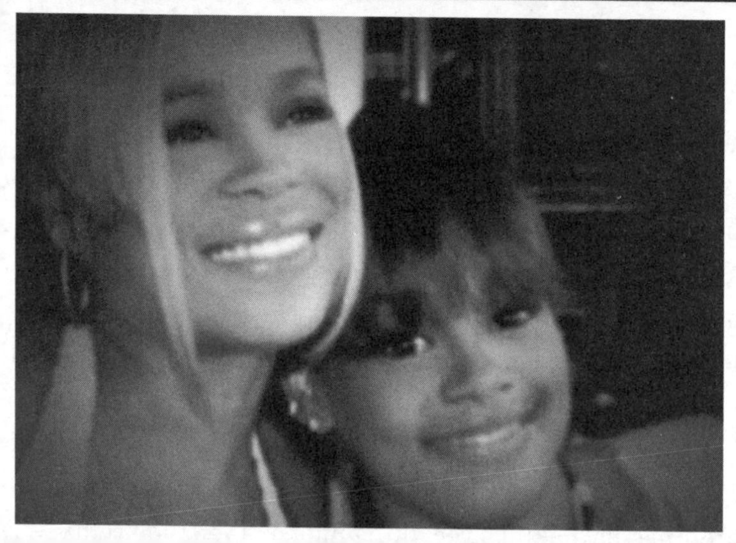

I called Lisa by a lot of different names over the years because she had a lot of different personalities. Her middle name was Nicole, so sometimes I called her that. Sometimes it was Nicki, which was her wilder side, and sometimes LeLe, the shy girl. And, of course, she was Left Eye to the world. She was so many things, not just the persona that people on the outside saw. She was this force of nature. One day she was here, and then one day she wasn't.

After we'd finished promoting *FanMail*, I went into the hospital, struck down again by my disease. I was exhausted and sick, and there was an undeniable tedium that came along with being trapped inside the cold walls of a hospital for days on end. I had nothing to do but sit in the bed, waiting to feel better. Nurses constantly stuck me with needles, drawing blood and putting in IVs. Nurses have a bad habit of not listening, digging and tearing through your flesh with needle after needle, poking everything but your vein. My veins were so bad, totally blown out from all the IVs I'd had over the years . . . to the point that they put needles in my feet, breast, shoulders, neck or wherever the could find a vein. I wanted to get out of there so bad. I was convinced that my aunt's church group had hexed me, and that's why I was in the hospital.

My aunt had gotten in deep with this group of churchgoers, and one evening she invited me over to join one of their gatherings. They said they wanted to save my soul, which was crazy since I don't drink or do drugs nor have I done most of the things some of them had done in their own lives. They were judging me with no real knowledge. My aunt wasn't involved. She didn't realize what was happening. While she was outside, the group started laying hands on me and speaking in tongues and praying, saying things like "She's sleeping with the enemy." They were referring to my husband. It was crazy. I got out of there quick, not even saying goodbye to my aunt.

After I left, I felt really weird and I had pain on my left side. I had to leave a recording session with Dallas to go to the ER, and as soon as I walked into the waiting room, I told my cousin Marde, "I'm not going to leave here for a while." I really felt it. After being hospitalized for 2 weeks, they tried to send me home. My blood work didn't match what I was telling the doctors I was feeling. I went home and passed out in the bathroom.

You can be sick and sometimes your body reacts to the pain first, before any real results show up in medical tests. Some doctors think they know it all and don't listen. But there was something majorly wrong with me. I ended up having pleurisy, which is fluid in my lungs, a dying spleen, and pancreatitis, as well as one of my usual sickle cell crises. My veins refused to cooperate, so the doctors were forced to put a triple lumen in my neck to connect to my artery. I had one cord to draw blood out, one to administer medicine, and a third to feed me intravenously because I couldn't drink or eat real food. It was terrible. I was bummed out and convinced I was hexed and stuck for what ended up being 4 months.

When you're in the hospital, anything helps. Any connection from the outside world, any reminder that people were thinking of me made a difference. It helped to take my mind off what was going on. The most important person and the best medicine for me is my mom, but I'd like support from my friends, too. Lisa knew that because she'd watched me go in and out of hospitals so often. Things had been so tense, and she was still angry at me for dissing her music with Suge Knight, but I never stopped caring about Lisa or our friendship.

During this particular hospital visit, Lisa sent me plants and letters every day for several days. Each one felt like a small motion to mend the cracks between us. "Get better," she wrote. "I'll be waiting for you." The plants began to line the windowsill of my room, slowly brightening it.

On the third day, a package arrived. I peeled back the paper and found a drum cymbal. On it, in black ink, Lisa had scrawled a picture of a clock on it and written, "Take all the time you need." It meant that I shouldn't worry if my disease was keeping the band from doing something, that my illness wasn't an inconvenience. She was giving me permission to heal.

On my fourth day, I didn't get a plant or a package or a letter. Instead, I heard Lisa's voice soaring through the hospital hallway. She was so loud. I loved that about her.

"Tionne," she exclaimed, bursting into my room. I knew she was there to apologize. She was leaving the next day to go to Honduras, and she wanted to make sure we were cool.

We were, somehow. That's the power of a friendship like ours, that you can forgive and forget as quickly as things can fall apart. It was like we'd never fought, like things had never fallen off track. That was unspoken between us. We just smiled and hugged and that said it all. It didn't feel significant in the moment—it was just another bump in the road that we'd overcome. I had no idea that was the last time I'd ever see Lisa.

Lisa wanted a break from TLC and a break from her life at home. She'd struggled through the process of *FanMail* and in her solo endeavors, and I think she couldn't quite pinpoint who she wanted to be going forward. She went back to Honduras in search of herself. She'd been going to Honduras a lot over the past few years to work with a man named Dr. Sebi, an herbalist. She stopped eating meat and sugar and was constantly on a cleanse. She was trying to find religion, and she also got into numerology. I had tried some of the herbs Dr. Sebi recommended, to see if it could help with my sickle cell. It didn't work for me. I have to be careful with certain herbs. I ended up in the hospital with another crisis after taking them. But to me this trip didn't seem strange—it was just what Lisa did.

She filmed the trip, which later became a documentary called *The Last Days of Left Eye.* In the footage, she said she had premonitions. She felt like a spirit was chasing her. She'd gotten in a car accident while her assistant was driving, and they'd unintentionally killed a small boy. She thought the spirit accidently killed him instead of her because his last name was Lopes, too. She took care of all his funeral expenses. She had a big heart. I felt as though she should have ended the trip then, but they stayed on. We weren't really in touch while she was away. I was still in the hospital, dealing with my own life and trying to survive because my organs were failing, and she was on this journey. I knew she'd come back and we'd be cool and we'd go back into the studio and work again.

On April 23, 2002, I was out of the hospital. I was frail and weak, and I'd dropped so much weight. I weighed 92 pounds. I was skin and bones. I felt like an elderly old woman, skin sagging off my legs. I had to go to the doctor every Tuesday for a year afterward just to be sure I was okay. My spleen was so fragile that the doctors told me that if I wore a seat belt and the car stopped suddenly, it could rupture and I could die.

I was feeling well enough to go to my cousin Marde's birthday party on the 25th, even though I'd been out only a few days. I bought a house in Atlanta, and sold the one in California at the time, and I was glad to be in Atlanta now because it meant I could see my family. I leaned against the window of my Porsche as my security guard Dave drove me across town to the party. But something felt off.

"Stop," I said. I was having a premonition of my own. I was certain that I was going to get in a crash. "We have to go back and switch cars," I told him.

"Why?" Dave asked.

"I feel like I'm going to get in a wreck," I told him. I felt so sure of it.

"You don't ever seem nervous like this," he said. He thought I was tripping.

"I don't know," I replied. I had this crawling feeling at the back of my neck. "I just feel like something is going to happen to me."

So he drove me all the way back home and we climbed into my Hummer instead. That thing was like a tank. It felt so much safer. We were okay to drive back to party. But that premonition wasn't about me, as it turned out. My car, no matter which one I drove, wasn't ever going to crash.

That evening, I came home from the party and put Chase to bed. I settled in the rocking chair in her room to watch *Judge Mathis* while she slept. At around midnight, my phone rang. It was Chilli. She was weeping so hard I could barely understand what she was saying.

"It's Lisa," she sobbed, struggling to get the words out. "She's been in a wreck." I didn't understand what that meant.

"What?" I asked.

"Lisa is dead," Chilli managed. She'd heard it from our manager. I didn't know how to process the information at all. I hung up and just stood there, immobile. The first stage of grief is denial, and that's a real thing. As I stood there, suddenly Chase bolted awake and starting screaming. It was like she knew. It was like she felt whatever I felt. I'd dealt with death before and it's always painful, but not like this. You're somewhat prepared for death if you know someone is sick with cancer or going to die, but never for unexpected ones. If someone is sick, you have enough time to grapple with the idea of loss.

I ran downstairs to tell D'mon, tears pouring down my cheeks, holding my screaming baby. This time I knew it was real—it wasn't one of Lisa's tricks. I wished it was fake. I knew it was true because of the way the phones went off when Aaliyah died; my phone started going off the same way. It wasn't a bad joke. This time it was true.

We quickly found out what had happened: Lisa had been driving a car in Honduras, and it had gone off the road. There were seven other people in the car, but she was the only one who didn't survive the crash. The reports said Lisa had been speeding and lost control. The car had rolled and she'd died from head trauma instantly. Four of the other passengers had to be hospitalized. Lisa had died at the same time I had decided to switch cars. My premonition had been about her.

By 4:00 a.m. we had to release a statement about Lisa's death to CNN. "We had all grown up together and were as close as a family," the statement said. "Today we have truly lost our sister." We didn't know what else to say. What are you supposed to say in a situation like this? There really are no words.

The day the news broke was my birthday. Lisa died on April 25, and the next day was my birthday. I spent the day at her mom's house, and there was nothing to celebrate. After we arrived at the house, Lisa's mom saw me and Chilli sitting together and almost fainted because she didn't see her daughter with us. It was too much for her to bear to see TLC with a member missing. Pebbles came over, too. We hadn't seen or spoken to her in a long time. She'd recently found God, so she kept trying to put prayer cloths over our heads and force us to lie down and confess our sins and get healed. She was what I call a baby Christian. Baby Christians are people who find God midway through life and think they know more than most because they have this newfound thing they're so deep into. I grew up with faith. I went to church my whole life. I didn't need this right now. Finally I told Dallas, "Just lay back so she'll stop." We all pretended to let her heal us so she'd go away and let us grieve in peace. Maybe she was sincere. But it was the wrong time to get us to confess our sins.

The news was everywhere. It was front-page stuff, and the

world was crying with us. Chilli and I were asked to call in to MTV's *TRL* to talk about what had happened. We didn't want to, but it felt like our duty to our fans. John Norris, whom we'd known for years, opened the show by announcing the news of Lisa's passing. Then he got us on the phone. Chilli was sobbing hysterically. Neither of us was prepared to do this.

"If one of you feels up to talking, can you tell us how you found out this happened?" John asked. Chilli was crying too hard to speak.

"Yes," I said. "This is T-Boz."

"How were you guys informed of what happened?" John asked.

I took a deep breath. "I heard it from Chilli, who heard it from our manager first," I said. I tried to remain as calm as possible. Thousands of fans were listening right now.

"Had you guys spoken to Lisa recently?" he asked.

I couldn't hold back the tears anymore. "I was in the hospital," I choked. "And that was the last time I'd seen her. I was in the hospital for 2 months, and she came to see me about 3 weeks ago."

John asked how Lisa was doing at the time. "She was doing good," I said. That was the truth. A few weeks ago, everything had been fine. "We were working on the album, but I got sick so we all kind of took a break so I could get better," I continued. "We all did our thing until it was time to go back into the studio."

"We had a lot of nice songs together," I added. We were supposed to be recording music with Lisa, not mourning her death. We'd been together for over 10 years. We were like sisters. I could barely get my head around it, even as I was on TV talking about it to the world. John asked us to share something about Lisa people might not have realized.

"Lisa had one of the biggest hearts of anybody we'd ever known," I said. "She would take a stray person off the street and give him the shirt off her back. She'd take all the money in her pocket and take care of whoever, whenever. She did charity work with kids all the time for lupus." I paused. "She was a very special person. Lisa could do anything she put her mind to."

We handed the phone over to our manager, who read a statement from Lisa's mom. As soon as I knew we were off the air, I collapsed into tears. No one should have to explain the death of their sister and bandmate on live TV. I knew then that nothing was going to be the same after that. Everything had changed when Lisa died. My whole world crumbled. We had something real, and that's what I'd loved about her. That day, as the news spread across the globe, was the end of TLC as we'd known it.

They flew Lisa's body back to Atlanta and funeral preparations began. It happened quickly. Her body arrived on a Monday and there was a memorial for her family on Wednesday. The wake took place in this funeral home. When the limo pulled up, I just sat there. I couldn't get out. My mom had to force me. It took 20 minutes because I felt like it would become real if I emerged from the limo.

Lisa's body was in a tiny room. I went in with my mom and D'mon and looked at her. She was lifeless. Tears ran down my face. As I was sitting there, I heard this voice next to me. "Bobbi!" she said. "Bobbi!" It was Whitney Houston. She had Bobbi Kristina, who must have been about 10 at the time, in tow. She dragged Bobbi Kristina up to me, as I was bawling my eyes out, and said, "You remember her? She knew you when you were in your mama's belly!" What was happening? I'm here crying over Lisa's body and Whitney's trying to tell her daughter how I knew her in the womb?

After I left the viewing, I crammed myself into this little holding room at the funeral home with Babyface, Chilli, Usher, Pebbles, Bobby Brown, Whitney, and D'mon. It was the size of a small closet, but somehow we were all packed in. Pebbles couldn't contain herself.

"See, Lisa should have came to me," Pebbles said. "I could have saved her."

Excuse me? No. She couldn't have saved her. This was what had happened. There had been eight people in the car, and Lisa was the only one who didn't make it. It was her time. No one wants to hear that when a loved one has passed away. If that's what was meant to have happened, it would have. I believe everything happens for a reason, even if we don't like or understand the reason.

"Babyface, me and you used to talk every day," Pebbles said next, oblivious to the situation around her. "Usher, you bought my house and I don't ever see you. We got to do better than this."

I couldn't process this. It was too much. I was 92 pounds because I'd spent 4 months in the hospital. I looked like a toothpick. My eyes were red from crying. D'mon took my hand and pulled me out of the room. "You just got out of the hospital," he said. "And you don't need all this drama. Let's go."

The actual funeral took place the following morning at the New Birth Missionary Baptist Church in Lithonia, Georgia. Thousands of people showed up. Literally, thousands. MTV claimed it was close to 10,000 fans, but I have no idea. It was a blur. Some of the fans had traveled miles to be there, and they arrived with posters and hand-painted portraits of Lisa. A lot of artists came to pay their respects, too. Usher, Janet Jackson, Whitney, Bobby, Monica, Suge Knight, Babyface—all there.

The service lasted 2 hours, everyone crammed into the church. They played a video montage of Lisa, and L. A. Reid, Lisa's brother Ronald, and her aunt Pamela all spoke. Her mom read a poem she'd written for Lisa before her death. Mary Mary, one of Lisa's favorite groups, played. The entire funeral was one of the most surreal experiences of my entire life. It obviously wasn't funny at the time, but when I recall it now, it seems like something out of a bad sitcom. Fans were screaming and trying to take photos and videos. I thought, "This is not the time."

It was the longest funeral of my life. Lisa had been dating Suge Knight, and he fell asleep halfway through. He was actually snoring as the readings went on. Whitney and Bobby were seated behind me, and I am not exaggerating when I tell you that Whitney repeated every single word that the pastor said. If he said, "Thank you, Jesus," Whitney would croon, "Thank you, Jesus." She sung every word back out loud. I kept thinking, "This cannot be happening." But there was Whitney singing and rubbing my shoulder and saying, "It's gonna be all right, baby." At one point I turned around to look at Bobby and he just shrugged, acknowledging that she was acting crazy. But then 30 minutes later I looked back and he was hooping and hollering with her. It was a circus. When I think about it now, I can barely believe it was real. I remember the antics of everyone there. Even the pastor—the notorious Bishop Eddie Long—seemed like he was putting on a show. He could have delivered a great speech. He just kept saying "watch this, watch this, watch this" like he was going to deliver some big, deep message, but he never did.

Lisa's casket had words from "Waterfalls" engraved in the wood. They read, "Dreams are hopeless aspirations, in hopes of coming true, believe in yourself, the rest is up to me and you." It was a good line and a hopeful one, too. The words and the casket and Lisa's body were laid to rest in the Hillandale Memorial Gardens in Lithonia. I missed her dearly and she was barely even gone.

It was impossible to move on after Lisa died. It was like no one would let us, either. The news was so big and she'd been so famous. Everyone everywhere was talking about her. I'd go to the movies and the people in the row in front of me would be chatting about her death. Or I'd go into a McDonald's and someone would say, "Did you hear about that girl Left Eye?" It was everywhere I went. Sometimes the people talking noticed me and sometimes they didn't. If they saw me, they'd just say, "Aww," or "Sorry about Left Eye." Others would offer condolences and then ask, "But can I take a quick photo with you?" Some would even tell me they could rap, like we were preparing to replace Lisa. It had been mere days since her death, and I didn't know how to take that. I couldn't tell if I was a real person to the fans. I couldn't tell if they recognized my pain and my grief, or if they just didn't care.

With this sort of stuff surrounding me, I become a hermit. I locked myself away. I'm not someone who's prone to depression. Who has time for that? But after Lisa died, I fell into a depression that lasted 2 years. Everybody has a breaking point. This was mine.

Lisa was my road dog and my creative partner, and she was gone. This became my reality. For 2 years I couldn't think about the creative stuff. It stopped making sense to me. It's not that I had no one to talk to about it, but I didn't want to constantly discuss it. No one knew what life on the road was like or what it meant to one of the world's biggest acts and to lose your third member while in the public spotlight. It was awful. I was so messed up. It was a life in TLC without the L. And a week after Lisa passed, I lost a good friend, the world-renowned makeup artist Kevin Aucoin. The stress took a toll on me. I ended up back in the hospital. I just lay there, sad. When you have children, though, you have to push through no matter what. You can't give in fully to the depression. I was heartbroken, but I still had a child to raise and feed.

Here's the thing about being an artist, too: Most people don't care if you're sad. There's a bottom line and people have to get paid. You've signed contracts. Albums have to be finished and released, and fans are waiting. If you have a sold-out concert, you have to go onstage and pretend to be happy, no matter what is going on in your personal life. You have to muster up the energy and keep on. Chilli and I worked through the grief because we had to. It wasn't an option to really feel our own sadness. The record label expected us to deliver *3D*, so that was what we had to do. We had to complete what we started with Lisa. The record label gave us some weeks off, but it didn't feel like enough. No amount of time would have been enough. And no matter how we were feeling, they expected an album. If you're an artist and you're unhappy, it shows in your work. I've had people ask me why I'm not a more sensitive person. This is why. Most people don't care, so you can't go around being fragile. You develop a thick skin because you have to.

We finished *3D*, and that album wasn't the best. I'm not

afraid to say it. There were a couple of good songs. One of them was "So So Dumb," which I wrote with Raphael Saadiq. Pharrell did one, which was cool. I wrote the first single, "Girl Talk," with Kandi Burruss, and I thought it was only okay. To this day, I don't want to perform it. Fans love it overseas because the beat is knockin' and it's fun to dance to. I knew I was slipping. I was under so much pressure. Lisa had died and I was being forced to finish an album I wasn't ready to finish. Even the album cover looks depressing. We look like death, wearing all black and frowning. I laugh about it now because Chilli's there looking like Batman and I have this face that looks like "Duhhhh." What were we thinking? Lisa was the only one who looked good, and she wasn't here anymore.

If I could go back, I would do it all differently. But we weren't in the right headspace to know. We just wanted to be left alone with our grief and have a little time off to heal. If we'd had more clarity, I think we would have released "Turntable" as the first single. I wrote it with Rodney Jerkins about Lisa's passing, and it was about how after something bad comes good. It talked about how all things happen for a reason. It would have given the album a different feeling and honored Lisa more, but it didn't occur to us to begin there at the time.

Lisa had left behind material she'd recorded for both *3D* and for her second solo album. We used three of her raps, and took some of her vocal recordings to help flesh out the material. But it wasn't the same. It wasn't like having her there to write new lyrics or to be with us in the studio. Her style before she passed was somewhat poetic. We needed to match the vibe of her lyrics and raps to our music, and a lot of it didn't fit. Our music just wasn't like that. Plus, Suge owned the gangster rap stuff she made as N.I.N.A., and no one wanted to deal with him. It was never even an option for us to replace her. That wouldn't have been right or felt right. We did the best we could with what was left. We wanted, at least, to pay tribute to Lisa.

The best memory I have of *3D* is Chase there in the studio with me the entire time. She was not even 2 years old, and she was more attached to me than usual. She refused to be away from me, even in the next room. She got really clingy after Lisa died, like she could feel the sadness, and she spent every minute of the album sitting on my hip. You can hear her crying on the Missy Elliott and Timbaland song because she came with me into the vocal booth. She was always connected to music because I sang to her while she was in the womb. I'd put speakers on my belly and played songs for her. After she was born, she seemed to find those songs familiar, turning toward the sound and cooing. Music is as embedded in my child's soul as it is in mine, so it feels right that she was part of making one of TLC's albums.

3D dropped on November 12, 2002, 7 months after Lisa's death. It was a hit immediately, landing at No. 6 on the *Billboard* 200 and eventually going platinum. I guess fans still cared—and some were at least curious. What would TLC be like without Lisa? We got positive reviews. *Billboard* said the album seemed like a fitting tribute to our fallen sister, which felt good to hear. We shot all of the music videos without Lisa. At the end of the "Girl Talk" video, we ran a tribute to her, leaving fans with the words, "In Loving Memory of Lisa 'Left Eye' Lopes."

We ended up getting two Grammy nominations for *3D*, despite my personal feelings about its quality. Chilli and I went to the awards show to represent. We smiled on the red carpet and waved to the press. We wore glittering diamond belts on our black pants that paid homage to Lisa, each one depicting the words *Left Eye*. We emblazoned our pants and jackets with giant white eyes. I even had her symbols on my earrings. Everything we wore was about her. Joan Rivers interviewed us as we made our way into the show.

"Do you think you'll add a third member to the group?" she asked us.

"Never, never, never, never," Chilli said, shaking her head. "You can't replace a TLC girl."

"So how do you do it?" Joan asked. "How do you change the arrangements when there are three of you?"

"Actually," I said, "we were done with more than half of the album before she passed on. So we're just keeping this album going and then we'll see what happens. But no, it's the same." I felt myself pulling back. "It's the same," I repeated. But it wasn't, exactly, and we all knew it. Everything was going to be different now.

We didn't win anything that year, but it didn't matter. We were still a band, no matter what, no matter who was missing. We wanted the world to see that TLC was still standing. But what now? Chilli and I needed a break from the band. We needed to heal and figure out who we were without Lisa. I was going to have to just be Tionne for a while and find out what my world would look like without my group.

CHAPTER 10

Life Without TLC

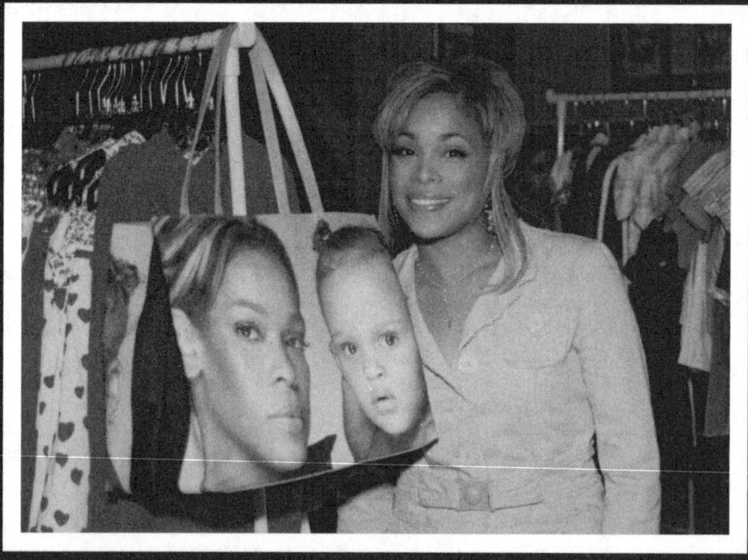

After Lisa died, a lot of people stopped believing in TLC. It was a strange phenomenon. The industry and the fans associated the three of us together, so it was hard for people to imagine that we could continue on with only two. People always viewed TLC as one. After Lisa burned down Andre's house, I'd been forced to prove to everyone that I wasn't an arsonist, too.

We were three separate people, and sometimes, I think, people had a hard time realizing we had separate lives, too. Record label execs, including LA, counted us out. How would TLC perform? How could we make it? Questions were constantly flying around. But Lisa's passing didn't take away my talent. My talent didn't stop. TLC would never be the same, but we could adjust. We could create a new normal.

There was no talk of replacing Lisa. We shut down any supposition that would happen. But we knew that we could keep Lisa's spirit alive. She could live on in our style, our performances, our dances—everything. Each time we played a concert, her energy would be there. It might take time to get it all right, but TLC wasn't finished, and I wanted the world to stop discounting us.

In 2003, TLC played our first show without Lisa. It was in East Rutherford, New Jersey, at Giants Stadium, where we performed at the annual Z100 Zootopia radio concert. There were a ton of other artists there—Aerosmith, Mariah Carey, Ginuwine—and it felt strange to be getting back up on a stage in front of 60,000-plus fans. They billed the show as "TLC's final performance," although that's obviously not what it was. It was a great way to sell tickets, though. Britney Spears and Carson Daly came onstage to introduce us, and we opened the set with a video montage in dedication to Lisa. Chilli and I waited in the wings with our four backup dancers as the video clip rolled, emotions surging through us. I was nervous because I didn't want to let the crowd down, but I also didn't want to cry in front of them.

As we went onstage to perform, I forced myself to face the crowd. I didn't want to turn around because behind us was the giant video screen, covered in images of Lisa. The idea was that she was performing "Ain't 2 Proud 2 Beg" and "What about Your Friends" along with us. There was footage of the three of us together, which we still use in our shows today. It's changed some over the years, but it's there. It's meant to leave the crowd with a good feeling. That night, before we played "Waterfalls," Chilli told the audience, "This was Lisa's favorite song." Our set ended with "Waterfalls," which always feels sentimental regardless, and as we walked off, a photo of the three of us from our early years in TLC plastered itself up on the screen. I saw it out of the corner of my eye, and I knew nothing was going to be the same. It felt so impossibly hard, but we had to keep facing forward, both on the stage that day and in our lives.

Playing a concert without Lisa felt surreal. It was like I was floating out of my body, watching something I couldn't connect to completely. I was numb. I felt like all of my moves and my lyrics were programmed into me and I was a robot who just had to do what I was put up there to do. I had to show people we could perform without our third group member. Onstage, I was emotionless. I always enjoy the fans, but there was a void. I looked forward and I sang and I danced, and we were still TLC. This was hard and it was going to take a long time for it to get any easier. Some nights were easier than others. You never knew which emotions would hit. On some days, I'd just break down and cry.

There was never any internal discussion that TLC would break up, despite how challenging it felt. Chilli and I didn't want the band to end. We blindly kept moving forward. After we played the show in New Jersey, it was clear that Chilli and I needed to take some space to heal. I didn't entirely know what that would mean for me. I'd been part of this group for years now. I'd gotten used to life on the road and in the studio with them. We spent more time with each other than our own families. It was weird to be without them.

Chilli and I continued doing things with TLC that weren't concerts. We did an awesome campaign with Pfizer to promote a new drug they had for AIDS patients. It had nothing to do with music. We had no current plans to make any new music. We still had bills to pay and kids to feed. I spoke solo at seminars about sickle cell. It was a difficult time. My personal life had started to crumble, as well.

I was a mother and a wife outside of the band. But all was

not well on the home front. D'mon and I were not happy. We stopped making sense together. It's important to know when you've outgrown something and when it's time to leave. I had to face that truth. On June 8, 2004, I filed for divorce. Chase was 3 years old at the time.

Everyone loves drama, especially when it involves someone famous, so it can be easy to forget that celebrities are real people. The press had a field day with it. It was heartbreaking, the same way it is when any couple calls it quits. The media likes to ignore that fact, but I was hurting—a lot. The press didn't have their facts right, either. I never said anything bad about D'mon to the press. It's not their business anyway, and I would never hurt my daughter or his children like that. Things got really messy, and I think what happened between the two of us should remain behind closed doors.

I learned a lot about myself during the divorce. Going through that process taught me so much. I learned what I should and shouldn't do in any future relationship. I learned to keep things to myself. It doesn't always make sense to reveal the drama between two people to your families, because it can come back to bite you in the ass. Don't drag other people into your mess. I've always felt I didn't need a man to be happy, but when you're going through a breakup, you second-guess yourself. Change is never easy!

Being married and moving in with D'mon had been a serious adjustment for me. I wasn't used to shacking up. I'm a very affectionate person, and when I love someone, I love hard, but I think it's also okay to miss someone. You can take time for yourself. I'm not the type of chick to be under someone 24/7. That would wreck my nerves. Some of us hopefully learn that lesson after being in a few relationships—I know I did. You have to step back and see what it is you really want and need from companionship, and be honest with yourself while doing so. Raising kids can be hard, too, depending on the difference in your values and your upbringing.

I thought we were ready to be married; I don't think we really were. The night before the wedding, when I was pregnant, I was so unsure. I didn't know if I should go through with it. I remember asking my cousin Marde if I was making the right choice, and she said it was probably just my hormones making me wonder. But then I think that everything happens for a reason. Life brought me D'mon, and we stuck it out for as long as we could. Maybe I was supposed to go through all that to learn about myself and what I need. Being a wife was one thing, but being a mother taught me the true meaning of love! There's no love like it.

No one is all good or all bad. Even if things didn't work out between me and D'mon, I still could see his good qualities. No matter how it ended, I don't regret our marriage. He gave me Chase, my greatest accomplishment, and after all that, I became an even stronger woman.

Here's something else I learned watching so many other women dealing with relationships: You should never stay with someone if it's not right or just for the kids. Don't let anyone treat you less than you deserve. You're worth more than that. Sometimes we settle because we're afraid to be alone or because we are afraid of change. But you shouldn't shack up for the sake of shacking up. I don't believe in playing house. Have you heard the term "Why buy the cow if you can get the milk for free?" You should never move out of state for a man with no hardware on your finger—I wouldn't. It takes a lot of years to really know who you are as a person and to know what you need on a daily basis, and know the same about someone else. It takes trial and error to find that out.

If a relationship feels off or you're not getting your just due, move on. There's going to be someone else out there worthy of you. Sometimes people are afraid to be alone, but you can do bad by yourself. It can be good to heal and let go of old baggage. You can survive without a man. When I was fresh out of my marriage, I told myself that I could do this solo, even if it meant being a single mom. The most important thing is my happiness and the happiness of my child. Was it hard or scary at times? Heck yeah! But I always face my fears.

You can't change people, which is something I learned dealing with my dad, and you need to learn to accept people for who they are and how they are. It's up to God to fix whatever needs fixing. People can heal and forgive. I'm not mad at D'mon and he's not mad at me. He loves Chase and my son Chance, and that's all that matters.

The divorce was hard for me, and it was harder because we were in the spotlight. I felt like I wasn't standing on solid ground most of the time. But there's a lot you learn when life drops a series of bombs on your head. I had to figure out what I was meant to do with the rest of my life. I knew TLC wasn't over, but for now we were paused. I'd missed out on a lot of solo opportunities because I'd given so much time to TLC. Sometimes I wonder what my career would have been if I'd put TLC on hold instead. I struggled to find artistic inspiration. Some artists, when they get depressed and heartbroken, feel the urge to create. I didn't. I missed Lisa, and it didn't feel right making music without her. So I had to decide, what was I going to do?

I pushed myself to record a solo album. I did it because I thought people expected it of me, not because it felt natural. I had an offer on the table from L. A., but he was fired, so that was the end of that. I needed something else, maybe something unrelated to music.

If I hadn't been a singer, I was going to be a fashion designer. That was the only other career that ever really interested me. I've always loved style. I used to dress TLC for some of our early photo shoots and videos. I'd fly to New York, shop on LaFace's dime, and pick out our outfits. Style and fashion was something that felt familiar.

When Chase was 2, I spent $78,000 in a single year on her clothes. She was so well-dressed. I bought her Prada, Roberto Cavalli, Miss Blumarine, D&G Jr., and Louis Vuitton. She was one of the first babies to ever wear Juicy Couture when it came out. Whatever was hot, she wore.

Thanks to Jennifer Bandier, the ex-wife of our manager, Bill, for introducing me to all the expensive baby stores. She and I got really close, and she took me to this high-end children's clothing shop called Z'Baby, where Tara Brivic-Rowntree worked as a stylist and personal shopper. The first thing Tara said to me was, "Okay, I am so happy your baby came out pretty 'cause I just don't think your husband's that hot." I busted out laughing. I dropped thousands of dollars at Z-Baby thanks to Tara and Jennifer. But the connection also inspired me. If there's one constant in this world, it's that people are always going to have babies. And they're always going to need to dress their babies. I could be part of that.

In 2004, Tara and I opened a store called Chase's Closet in the River Oaks Shopping Center in Houston (which is basically the Rodeo Drive of Houston). The shop, which I had designed to look like Chase's actual closet, sold children's clothes for both boys and girls, ranging from infants to 12-year-olds. At first I'd wanted to open the shop in Atlanta, but it was too costly. Tara had recently moved to Houston and suggested we try it there instead, and it ended up feeling like the right spot. The idea was that we stocked only a couple items per size for every style because we wanted the kids to feel like little individuals. To me, style wasn't about looking like everyone else or following a trend—it was about finding your own way of expressing your personality through your clothes. I wanted kids to feel that way, too. They could be unique and special, instead of the same as everyone else.

It was such a personal project for me. It felt like a dream come true. It was so amazing to see my store come to life just as I'd imagined it. *People* listed us as one of the top 100 baby stores in America, and it was nominated for the number-one children's boutique in Texas for 4 years running. We also got a lot of celebrity connections. Angelina Jolie bought a shirt for her son Maddox, and we sold out of those shirts in a weekend just because he wore one. One of Julia Roberts's twins was photographed in another shirt and was on the cover of *US Weekly*. Solange Knowles shopped there. We had this VIP service where the store would send a box of clothes to you and you could send back anything you didn't want. It was a lot like the subscription boxes that are popular today, and it was meant to make the clients feel like they were getting a personal service without ever having to step into the store. We even took personal requests. We sent Paul Wall a blinged-out pacifier, which felt like the perfect fit for his child.

In TLC, aesthetics had always been key. We'd been famous for our style. First Lisa stuck that condom over her eye; then we embraced baggy pants, giant, colorful shirts, and Cross Colours. Clothes are meant to be fun. They tell a story. Our look evolved over the years, but I think the consistent thing was that we made it our own. No one dressed like us, and they still don't to this day. They've tried to rip us off, but we were the original. Female singers today wear tiny little outfits even more so and take their clothes off a lot, but for us, the power was in the overall look, not how much of our midriffs were showing. We wanted to stand up for the chicks who didn't want to take their clothes off to prove they were sexy.

I also launched my own line called Chase's Closet during the store's 4-year tenure. One of my dresses, the Chaser, was featured in *Child* magazine. Every dress sold really well. I felt like I had created something meaningful again, even if it wasn't music. It was a relief to know that I still had the drive and ability to create. It's something I'm continuing to pursue now, designing a line of children's clothes called Baby Bouge, and while I am inherently a performer, it's nice to express myself in other ways, too.

By 2005, I'd settled into my life more. I had my store and I was finding inspiration there. The divorce was final. Every morning I'd wake up and remember what a miracle Chase was and how lucky I was to beat the odds. Although TLC wasn't ready to make any new music or go back on the road, the band did resurface for a while. UPN came up with this idea to create a reality show around TLC where Chilli and I searched for a person to perform with us to see what the TLC experience was like. The show, *R U the Girl?*, was never meant to replace Lisa, although some people got confused about that. The winner of the show would get to sing with us on a new single, but they weren't going to become a part of TLC.

UPN started a casting call in February of 2005, going around the country looking for semifinalists to be on the show. Later, they filmed me and Chilli around New York,

Miami, LA, and Atlanta, visiting the semifinalists and delivering the news that they'd been offered an opportunity to audition for us. To be honest, a lot of the reason I did the show was because it was a nice payday. I got a big chunk of money, and the show was generally a success, but I didn't want to be there. I put on a happy face for the cameras.

People kept asking, "Oh, so you're replacing Left Eye?" We weren't. We never said we were. Everyone heard us say "We're not replacing Lisa" over and over. They heard it from the horse's mouth, and they still didn't believe us. It was frustrating. I still didn't really know how TLC should be without Lisa. I felt like I was constantly trying to prove that we would be okay and that we could continue on. There was no talk of another album yet, though. Chilli and I weren't ready. I still had other things on my agenda as Tionne, rather than T-Boz. I even got offers like being in *People*'s Most Beautiful People issue—twice.

I knew my story was unique for a lot of reasons. Dallas Austin and I always reflected on our time at Jelly Bean's. It was such a singular place. It had this unique vibe, and it meant so much to everyone who grew up in Atlanta during that time. We talked for years about making it into a movie. I joined forces with Jody Gerson to finally pitch it, basing it on Dallas's and my story of growing up in Atlanta and dancing at a skating rink. I knew Jody because she gave me my first publishing deal at EMI. She told me, "You have the talent to write." She helped me believe in myself and to find my inner writer. She had a lot of connections to movie producers and studio executives, so she was the perfect person to put this movie in motion.

We approached producer James Lassiter, who was Will

Smith's partner at Overbrook. I pitched him on the idea in his office with Dallas. I acted an entire scene out. "This how we used to dress," I explained, motioning. "This is what we used to do. I don't have a script, but this is how I see the movie." He smiled. He got exactly what I was envisioning and agreed to help us.

Chris Robinson, who's directed music videos for people like Jay-Z and Alicia Keys, took it on as his first film. He was the right fit because he could capture both the music aspect and the story. Chris and Dallas spent a bunch of time together in Atlanta so he could get the right vibe of the city. There was talk of shooting scenes in New Orleans or Canada, but Dallas and I refused. It had to be made in Atlanta.

Dallas coordinated all the music for the film. The idea was that *ATL* would tell an emotional coming-of-age story that captured the feeling of Atlanta and Jelly Bean's during that era. We ended up getting T.I. to play the lead, which was amazing because it was his first time acting in a movie. Big Boi, Killer Mike, and Monica all made appearances. Lauren London played me—or, rather, a version of me. Her character wanted to dance with the guys, just like I had. The only difference was that me and Dallas never dated in real life.

We shot *ATL* over the summer in 2005, and it was a great experience for me. I couldn't be on the set as often as I wanted to because TLC had to promote *R U the Girl?*. Yet again, the band took me away from a personal project I was passionate about. It took me 11 years to get this movie made, and I couldn't even be there to see the entire thing through.

ATL came out on March 31, 2006, and came in third at the box office that weekend. Critics liked it, for the most part, and the movie got nominated for a few awards, including an

NAACP Image Award. It even won Best Hip Hop Movie at the BET Hip Hop Awards in 2006. There was controversy attached to it, too. Some theaters refused to screen it because it was "too urban." They called it an "urban black movie" and said that encouraged gang violence just because T.I. was in it. But it wasn't that sort of film. It had a positive ending, and it was about finding yourself. T.I. is supposedly working on a sequel, but I'm not involved. Telling my story in *ATL* was enough to satisfy me.

The years passed and Chilli and I didn't really discuss making another TLC album. We kept pursing our own lives and our families. We started to heal. I found out who I was outside of the band at the time and what I wanted in the future. Little did I know that the trials and tribulations weren't over. Life had another giant hurdle in store for me.

CHAPTER 11

Mind Over Matter

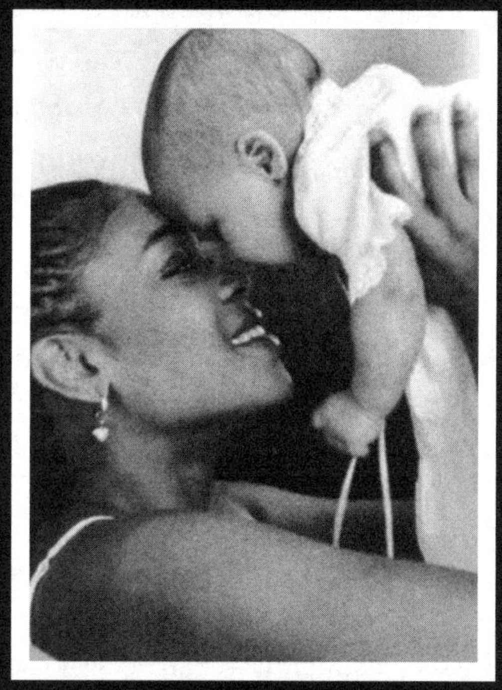

After Lisa died and after my divorce, everything was a struggle. Gravity felt stronger than usual, pushing down on me. My body fought itself constantly. When I get emotional, my disease flares up more than usual, and this time was no different. As all these bad things happened, as I tried to deal with my grief and cope with the loss of my friend and my husband, I had good months and bad months.

Sometimes it was like I wasn't even sick at all, but then I'd collapse and wind up back in the hospital. To make matters worse, I tore my meniscus and my cartilage started thinning. It was yet another ailment I had to work to maintain. Plus, wherever your body is weak in the first place, the sickle cell pain goes.

I got an ear infection that spread into my bloodstream that required surgery and a week in the hospital. Then I got the Norwalk virus and almost died. My mama found me passed out in my closet and forced me to go to the hospital.

Where did I even get the Norwalk virus? That's something you find on ships, and I hadn't been on any ships. I was a mess, clearly. It felt like I had a long road to recovery ahead of me.

Then, in the fall of 2007, I started getting excruciating headaches. Yet another thing wrong with my body. I thought it was stress. I went to get massages and acupuncture, trying to help ease my pain. But the headaches became too severe. I became too dizzy to even stand. I knew something was wrong. I kept thinking, "Oh my God, what else?" Finally, after weeks of pain, my mama said, "Go to the doctor. Get it looked at."

They gave me an MRI, but it takes several days to get those results back. So I waited. I was used to waiting for tests to come back. I was in a boutique owned by Bow Wow's mom Teresa, shopping with my friend Gail, when Dr. Braunstein, the doctor who usually helped me with my sickle cell, called. I pressed the talk button. "Hello?" I said, standing next to a rack of shirts.

"Tionne, where are you?" he asked.

"I'm out shopping." I flipped through the shirts.

"Go home and call me back." Dr. Braunstein sounded serious. But I wasn't prone to panic, not after all these years. Whatever he had to say, he should say now. Bad news is bad news no matter where you are, although I was definitely getting tired of hearing it.

"Tell me what you have to tell me now," I said. I figured it was something serious or he wouldn't want me to go home first, but I wanted to hear it now. I blurted, "Do I have a brain tumor or something?"

He went quiet. There was a moment of stillness. I dropped

the shirt sleeve. Panic crept in, slowly. I had said it not really knowing if I meant what I said. Finally he replied, "You do have a brain tumor."

The news punched me in the face. I felt the tears start falling down my cheeks. I couldn't focus on anything else my doctor said to me. He kept talking, but it was gibberish, background noise. Was this real? What was happening? After everything, now this?

He hung up. I think I said goodbye, but I don't remember. I was still in the store, next to some shirts I didn't want. I caught my breath and dialed my mama straight away. She was in Des Moines, with so much distance between us. I was desperate to talk to her. But she didn't answer. The phone just rang and rang and I mumbled out a message. "Mama, call me back right now." Where was she?

I walked out onto the sidewalk. I had no interest in shopping now. Gail took me across the street to eat at my favorite Mexican restaurant to cheer me up. I didn't have a choice but to carry on with my day. I might have a brain tumor, but I still had to eat lunch. I tried calling my mom again on the way over. No answer again.

I wondered, "How much tragedy is enough for one person?" In a perfect world, we'd all get a certain amount of hardship and sorrow and then we'd tap out, free and clear. But life isn't fair. Some people are given more to deal with than others.

By the time my mama called me back, I was finished with lunch and back in the car. I answered the call and came out with it.

"Mama, I have a brain tumor," I said. The words sounded so unbelievable as they fell out of my mouth. Not even real. I started crying again. Something about talking to your mother makes you feel like a child again. I just wanted her to make it all better. My mom, always calm, told me we would figure this out. That's what moms say when something bad happens. It's what I say to my daughter. But was it going to work out this time? I didn't really know.

When we hung up and I went home, my house felt empty and alien. I had this sense like I was falling and trying to grab hold of something on the way down, but there was nothing to grab. It was hard to focus on the truth and just accept it outright. I thought about how I'd hauled around a lot of sadness and worry throughout the years. Had I been burdened with more than my share? Of course, those sorts of thoughts don't help. Life gives you what it gives you, even when it's something you don't understand, and you can only go on from there. I allowed myself one day to sob and then I decided to fight, just like I've always fought through everything else.

The next few days were the longest of my life as I waited for appointments to find out what exactly was in my head. I started thinking in circles. Was I going to die? Was it cancerous? What would happen to my daughter? On the fourth day, I finally made it in to see a series of specialists to get a real diagnosis. Dr. Braunstein had given me his opinion, but since his specialty isn't neurology, we all wanted to be sure we knew what was going on.

After a series of appointments, the diagnosis arrived. I had a rare brain tumor called an acoustic neuroma. It was the size of a grape and nestled deep in my right cerebellum behind my ear, pressing on my facial, hearing, and balance nerves. It was bad. It was a dangerous location for a tumor because it could affect so much. I could lose my hearing. I could lose my balance. My face could become distorted and affect my sight. I could become so dizzy the world would feel like it was constantly spinning—as if the world isn't already spinning enough.

I wanted to ensure that I found the right person to deal with this. It needed to be the right surgeon, not just someone who saw me as a task or a dollar sign. I'm the type of person who goes on vibes and gut feelings. I won't just trust anyone. I needed a doctor who would try everything in his or her power to save me, and it seemed like no one wanted to do that. I saw a ton of doctors in Atlanta, but my gut kept telling me that none of them were the right person.

Everyone told me that there were two options to handle the tumor. They could treat the tumor with radiation and leave it in my head, which wasn't a long-term option. It wasn't a real cure because it meant continuing to deal with the tumor for the rest of my life. It also involved burning away brain tissue, so you could come out with no memory and a tumor still inside your head, possibly deaf, dizzy, and blind with your face paralyzed, now or in years to come.

The other option was surgery to remove it. But the problem was that my body might not be able to handle that trauma because of the sickle cell. There was a possibility that my heart and lungs would collapse during the procedure and fail. Some of the doctors said that old-school surgery wasn't a good idea for me because of my age and my disease. So neither option was great—and neither sounded good to me. The decision seemed impossible.

I struggled for days, asking my mama for advice and praying to God. After one of my doctor visits, my best friend Leslie went to get the car, and while my mama and I waited for him to pull it around, I noticed she was staring off into space.

"I wish it were me," she mumbled. I wasn't sure if she knew I heard her. I felt awful because of course I wouldn't trade places with her for the world. I've tried to put myself in her shoes. I couldn't imagine how I'd feel if it were Chase. But in the moment, it was hard to stomach my mother feeling that way. I could see the pain in her eyes. It gave me a reason to fight even harder.

It was hard, but we always found something to laugh at. During one appointment, my mama, Leslie, and I were meeting a new doctor. The doctor said, "Remember these words: green, circle, key. I'm going to ask you for them again in 15 minutes." She examined me, pushing on my head and looking in my eyes, to see what type of tumor I had. Fifteen minutes passed. I couldn't remember the words.

"Apple, grass," I began. Shoot. I listed off every word I could think of. None were right. My mom and Leslie were rolling. The doctor was worried.

"The tumor might be affecting her worse than we thought," she told us.

"Please," my mama replied. "This child's memory always been bad. The tumor didn't mess it up." I nodded. My memory had been tore up from the floor up since day one. It was a small moment during a lot of stressful moments, but it helped. It reminded us that we could still smile, even in the face of tragedy. Now, to this day, Leslie calls me "green circle key."

In the end, I decided I didn't want the tumor left behind. I wasn't going to leave some foreign thing in my head. It was better to take my chances on the surgery. I still had to find the right person to do this, though. I researched and researched, and two names kept coming up: Dr. Rick Friedman, an ENT-otolaryngologist, and Dr. Keith Black, a neurosurgeon. It was worth a shot. I got Dr. Friedman's cell phone number from someone and left him a message explaining the situation. He called me back from his son's baseball game.

At the time, my boyfriend was the NFL linebacker Takeo Spikes. His father had died from a cancerous brain tumor, so he knew about some of these doctors. You never know why certain people are brought into your life, but sometimes I wonder if Takeo was brought into my life for that reason. The timing of it was uncanny. Takeo sat on the call with me and Dr. Friedman, who was located in LA. I was living in Atlanta at the time, but I was willing to go wherever I needed to go to fix myself.

I had seen all these doctors in person and looked into their eyes, but I didn't feel the same way I felt about any of them as I did talking to Dr. Friedman on the phone. He was the guy. I just knew he was the guy. I knew it with such ferocity that I packed my bags and moved back to Los Angeles before I'd even met him face-to-face. When I got to LA and finally met him in his office, my instincts were confirmed. The doctor took my hand and looked me right in the eye.

"I will do everything in my power to save your life so you can have your career and be there for your daughter," Dr. Friedman confirmed. "The same way I would for my own family."

Tears poured down my face. I knew it. I knew he was the guy. He was going to save me. Dr. Friedman would work with Dr. Black and Dr. Gabriel Hunt, who is a spine specialist, on the surgery. They would go in the back of my skull and snip out the tumor. Dr. Black asked me to give him an order of preference for what I wanted to save. I picked my face first, because I needed it for my career, and then my hearing, because I'm a singer. I figured that if you looked at me, you wouldn't be able to tell if I was blind or deaf, so my face was the most important. I picked my balance last. They would do the best they could to save everything. At this point, I'd done all I could do and had to trust that this was going to work.

My family is amazing, especially during hard times. They came together to help me get things in order to prepare for surgery. Dr. Braunstein told me, "If you want to survive this, you need to get rid of all your stress." I had to block everything out. I had to ignore the press, who were still speculating on my divorce. I fired lawyers and assistants. I closed down my clothing store, Chase's Closet. I got rid of every person who could call me with any inkling of stress. I shut it all down. My family and close friends remained. They really stepped up, including my father, who came for the surgery. When he arrived, he had this look on his face like he was sorry for everything he'd done. I was glad for the support. It helped a lot.

I want to say a special thanks to Leslie, Marla, Shanti, Tia, Teliece, Wanda, Liz, my dad, Pastor Smith, Butch, and, of course, my mom. Thank you for praying for me and for being there by my side. My mom even had Chase's kindergarten class say a prayer for me because she said children's prayers are the purest. It really helped.

The day, November 7, 2007, arrived quickly. The night before the surgery, I lay in the hospital bed in Cedars-Sinai in Beverly Hills and ached to feel some peace. I was nervous. My lawyer had me sign power of attorney papers, and I'd taken out life insurance in case I didn't make it. The paperwork and my will made it feel all too real. And I knew my disease was going to make this surgery harder than it should be. I wanted to feel calm. I closed my eyes and asked God to release me from the fear.

"Whatever peace is, please give me that," I prayed. "Just make me not afraid." I wanted to believe that I would be okay because it seemed like the only way I'd survive.

The prayer worked. On the morning of the surgery, I felt at peace for the first time in my life. All my thoughts filtered out and my head went completely blank, and I felt nothing. I wasn't thinking about the possibility of dying or worrying about what might happen next. I was just quiet and still. The hospital staff thought I was nuts for having no emotions as they wheeled me into the surgery. But I was just calm. I was sure that God was listening.

The surgery lasted 7 hours. It wasn't supposed to be that long, but the tumor was rooted deeper than they'd initially thought. But they got it out.

The first thing I remember from waking up after the surgery is Takeo smiling and my aunt Wanda in the room. "Oh my God, you look so pretty," she exclaimed. "It looks like you have blush on your face. Your hair is still combed!" I was foggy because of the drugs, but I was happy to hear that my hair was untouched. It had been a long-running joke with the doctors that they weren't supposed to mess up my coif during brain surgery. "Who gets a craniotomy and thinks about their hairstyle other than you?" Dr. Friedman had said. But I didn't want them messing up my hairline.

As I woke up more fully, I heard Dr. Friedman whispering into my right ear.

"Can you hear me, Tionne?" he asked.

"Shh, I have to have surgery," I replied. I was so confused. But then I realized: He was testing my hearing and I could still hear. My ear still worked! They say if you come out of surgery looking okay, then most likely you'll end up with less or no paralysis. If you come out messed up, you'll stay messed up. So I thought everything was going to be fine because I looked fine and I could hear. Usually you have to do an MRI after and then go to the ICU, but I got to go back to my hospital room. That was a good sign, too.

After I got upstairs from the recovery room and the anesthesia wore off, the pain kicked in. I could suddenly feel that someone had been drilling into my skull. The trauma of the pain, which was immense, caused me to go into a sickle cell crisis that night. I had to stay in the hospital for 2 weeks. Everything hurt. And I don't really remember much. I woke up one day and my best friend Leslie was sitting on the edge of my bed, watching me. He looked like he was ready to catch a football.

"What are you doing?" I asked.

"I'm ready to catch you," he replied. "You've been flipping around across this bed. I don't know what drugs they got you on, but you're acting crazy."

I had to ask people to come to the bathroom with me. When you take so many pain meds, you can't pee or poop—it stops everything. I need people to sit there and talk with me and run the water. I would sit there for 2 hours before I could even pee. I started my period and I've never felt pain like that in my life, which is saying a lot for me. My legs had sharp, shooting pains running through them. Every single thing was magnified to the 10th degree. I legitimately felt like I was dying.

Recovering from brain surgery is one of the hardest things I've ever had to do—or for anyone to go through, whether you have sickle cell or not. It's a really long process that took me 3½ years in total. My surgery affected my balance, which I'll never get back, because they had to remove the nerve that controls the balance on my right side. During physical therapy, I was able to teach my left side to compensate 93 percent for my right side, but I still fall and trip sometimes. I only lost 3 percent of my hearing, which is miraculous. I could see again, although it was a little blurry.

I couldn't close my right eye for weeks after surgery. There are little things you take for granted, like blinking. You don't really realize how much you need your most basic bodily functions until they're taken away from you. I couldn't even blink. My eye had to be taped shut, and I had to put this greasy gel in my eye to help keep it lubricated. You could go blind if your cornea dried out. Eventually I got tired of taping it shut, so I would just hold my eye closed with my hand and sit there and watch TV. It was really uncomfortable. Everything felt more difficult than before.

After you have your skull opened up, they make you sit up for 24 hours a day for 2 months, which is impossible. If you lay down flat, fluid will fill your brain. My mom rigged every possible concoction to keep me upright while I slept. We bought everything the hospital had used while I was there. But I would still slide down every night. I ended up getting swelling in my brain and had to be hospitalized again. They were talking about cutting my head back open.

"No. I can't take anymore." I refused. "I don't think I'll make it through another one of these." I prayed about it a lot, and I got to go back home. It was touch and go all the time. A week after I got home from the hospital, I was eating pancakes and suddenly the bites of food fell out of my mouth. I lost everything, in a moment. I couldn't see. I couldn't hear. I couldn't talk. I looked at my mom crying, thinking, "What is happening?"

"Tionne," she said, "they told you this could happen."

Part of the process is that you can get worse before you get better. But at the time, there wasn't the technology to know exactly what was going to happen, so it was as much of a learning process for the doctors as it was for me. This particular situation was something that could happen to tumor patients before surgery, but I hadn't experienced it yet, which made it all that much scarier. I didn't imagine the healing process could go backward.

I gained a lot of weight from the steroids I had to take postsurgery. They had me on the highest amount of steroids possible, and I puffed up. I was taking over 30 pills a day. I went into the hospital as a size 4 and came out as a 2X, which seemed crazy. You go through a lot—mentally, physically, and emotionally—when your looks are affected. I felt like the swan who had become the ugly duckling. The press began talking about me. I saw myself in magazines and online with headlines that read, "T-Boz Gains 200 Pounds." It wasn't newsworthy, but everyone acted like it was. I could afford to lose weight, but I couldn't afford to lose my life—and I was sick, not fat. The world is so superficial and shallow to the point of carelessness.

When I looked into a mirror, I didn't recognize myself. I looked like the Elephant Man, so deformed. It hurt to see that reflected in the press and to feel like I had to be a hermit and stay inside. One day I caught my reflection and burst into tears.

"No," my mama said. "Stop that." I looked at her. "The doctor told you this is where you are now," she said. "It's a journey back to the other side."

She decided to take pictures of my face to show me my progress because I couldn't see it. I just felt swollen and messed up. My daughter, who was 7 at the time, didn't really understand what was going on. But Chase could see what I couldn't see, too.

One day she took both of her little hands and put them on my cheeks.

"Mommy," she said. "You're so pretty." I started crying. What in the world did she see that I couldn't? But it helped me decide that I would work to get better. I told Chase, "Mommy is going to be sick for a long time, and you've gotta help take care of Mommy. You have to make sure everybody is quiet." So she would go around telling people, "Shh, you have to be quiet. Mommy is resting." It was so cute. She brought me my food and sat and watched TV with me. She was the perfect little girl. My family really came through. You realize who's in your corner when you're sick like that. My mom, especially, was always there no matter what. It reminded me of the times we were broke growing up and she gave up her food so I could eat. She did whatever I needed to make me better.

It was my goal to make it home to Atlanta for Christmas. That was the absolute longest flight of my life. It was so painful. I had to be pushed around in a wheelchair, and I hoped no one would notice me. I wore these big shades to cover up my face, which was deformed and swollen. It was so painful with all the pressure up in the air. But it was worth it. I was so happy to see my own bed.

I started physical therapy in LA and continued it in

Atlanta. I had to relearn how to talk and walk again. They had me do all these simple exercises with video games where my eyes had to learn to refocus and follow images. I have a really long basement and took a deck of playing cards and taped them along each side of the wall. The idea was to walk straight and look to each side as I walked. It was horrible. I had so many bumps and bruises from knocking into the wall.

When we first started the physical therapy, I couldn't look left or right. I could barely sit in the car. It was hell riding to the doctor's office, which was only 10 minutes away, because I was so dizzy and it was so hard to focus. I finally got to the point where I could drive a car straight, but I couldn't turn my head around to back up. One day I wanted to prove to myself that I could drive around the corner to Blockbuster. But I couldn't back out. My mom was furious.

"You can't be doing this!" she shouted. "You know you can't see! You could have died!"

I was so stubborn and so bored. It's not fun being kept at home in front of a TV for that long when you're used to working. So I taught myself how to write movie scripts while I was idle. I had to do something to keep myself busy, so I figured I'd acquire some new skills.

But in the end, despite all the pain and frustration, I survived. If I'd had the surgery in Atlanta with the other doctors, I don't think I would have made it. I think I made the right choice for my body, and I credit that to doing all my research and searching until I found the right doctor. And I credit that to the fact that I decided I wanted to live.

When you've worked really hard all your life, it's hard to stop. Even though my body forced me to slow down and to reevaluate what I was capable of, it felt weird to slow down.

The recovery from my brain surgery happened in baby steps. And sometimes those steps went backward. But I wanted to work again. An opportunity came up to be cast on the second edition of NBC's *The Celebrity Apprentice*, which was then infamously hosted by Donald Trump. I decided to do the show before I was actually medically released by the doctors to do any work. I took it upon myself to do it because I wanted to prove to myself that I could get back into the swing of things.

The show shot in New York in the fall of 2008. We stayed in the Trump International Hotel & Tower, where I'd stayed with TLC several times before. I brought my mom and Chase along with me. Depending on how I did, the shoot could run for a month or two and I didn't want to leave Chase back at home. I had her homeschooled during the hours of shooting. The contestants were asked to pick a charity to donate their winnings to. I picked the Sickle Cell Foundation of Georgia, which had long been close to my heart thanks to Phil Oliver, and I genuinely hoped I could raise awareness and funds for the sick children. I'm always looking for ways to help other people with my disease, and this seemed like as good of an opportunity as any.

But when I got to New York, it quickly became clear this was all a mistake. It was the second time they'd done *The Celebrity Apprentice*, and the cast was notoriously diverse. Joan Rivers, Melissa Rivers, Khloé Kardashian, Dennis Rodman, Andrew Dice Clay—all there along with me. Some of the other people I'd never even heard of. I didn't care for Annie Duke. I'm not into hanging out with other celebrities. I thought Brande Roderick, who was a former Playboy Playmate, was pretty cool though. So was Natalie Gulbis, a professional golfer.

Filming was intense. The producers worked you 6 days a week, for 14 or 15 hours a day. They wanted to keep us sleep deprived. They kept us as hungry as possible. When food did show up, it was either cold or late. They wanted us to be irritable and pissed off so we'd get into it with the other contestants. Well, getting up at 5:00 a.m. always had me on the verge of being pissed off. On the first day, as I was leaving the hotel room, my mom said, "Tionne, you haven't ruined your career in 20 years. Do not go in there and fight with people and mess it up." I nodded. "Remember," she added, "you're there for a worthy cause." And I listened to her. No matter what happened, I kept my cool when the cameras were rolling.

On the first day, I had a temperature of 103. I had a bad cold and bronchitis, and I was barely hanging on. Dr. Primus, the hotel doctor on call, who I still use when I'm in New York, came to give me a shot of something. He wanted me to consider going to the hospital.

"No," I insisted, "I want to do the show."

On the first day, when everyone initially met me, I had to jump out of our van and vomit into a trash can on the street corner. It became clear pretty quickly that I was sick. Our first challenge was to make cupcakes and then sell them for more money than the other team. Joan was our team captain that day and we wanted to win. Because I was sick, I kept leaving the kitchen to go blow my nose and then wash my hands. I'd come back in the kitchen, wash my hands again, and continue to cook. It would have been nasty to deal with my cold while in the kitchen. So I wasn't being lazy; I was being clean. Annie acted like I was chilling in the hallway instead of working. But I worked really hard to get people to come down and buy those cupcakes.

I went on the radio and I got a bunch of TLC fans there. I got L. A. Reid to come down. He gave us $5,000. I brought in Steve Rifkind from Loud Records, who also gave us a $5,000 check. And I sold $4,000 in cupcakes on top of all that. I raised the third most out of my team, which was called Team Athena.

When we went into the boardroom, I was sitting in front of Melissa. Donald asked us who we thought the weakest link on the team was. "Tionne," Melissa said immediately. Um, what? I was sick, so I was just trying to get through the day. But if I hadn't have been sick, my response would have made it a totally different episode. I would have cussed her out right there in the boardroom. How could she say I was the weakest link? I was in third place for having raised the most money.

Outside, after he'd sent us away, she came up to me. "I didn't know what else to say when Donald asked me," Melissa tried to claim. "You were sitting in front of me, so I picked you."

I looked at her like, "Bitch, please." I don't respect that. You picked me because I was sitting there? That's stupid. There's eight people on this team and you say I'm the weakest link? And it's not like I hadn't known Melissa before this. She and I had been pregnant at the same time, and I'd been on an E! show with her. It's not like we were friends, but we'd been cool.

"You said what you said," I responded. "Whatever. It doesn't bother me." That crap rolled right off my back. I walked away as she was trying to explain herself because it was a waste of my time.

From that first day it pissed me off how people would just kiss Donald's ass. Whenever we went into the boardroom, they'd immediately switch from being cool into robots who'd be like, "Yes, whatever you say Donald Trump." I don't respect that. At the end of the day, he didn't have anything to do with my job. He couldn't stop me from eating. I didn't care who he was. I kiss no one's ass.

I was quiet on the show because I was sick and other women talking over each other gets on my nerves. I'm not actually quiet. So these heffas didn't know who they were messing with. I let it slide with Melissa. I didn't let her think I was sweating it. And I wasn't, really. But pick the person you really think is weak. Or if you think I'm weak, then say that. I was cordial to her after that, but I looked at her differently from then on.

I disliked Annie Duke most. She was so disrespectful to me. I had the flu, and I had all the symptoms that come along with the flu. When I had to leave the challenge a few times to blow my nose, Annie told Trump, "She kept leaving the challenge. She didn't do any work." Bitch, I was blowing my nose! I couldn't take it with her. She talked down to everyone. I waited until the cameras were off and then I cornered her.

"Look, Annie," I said. "I don't like the way you talk. I don't give a fuck how you talk to everybody else, but what you're not gonna do is talk to me that way."

She didn't seem to know what to say. "I'm just used to being a boss," she replied.

"I've been a boss my whole career," I said. "I was born a boss, boo." I paused, for effect. "Do you see your kids in this room?" I asked.

"No," she said.

"Exactly," I confirmed. "They're at home and I'm not one of them, so watch how the fuck you talk to me. What you're not gonna do is speak to me crazy." I was deadly serious. I think in that moment she realized, "Oh shit, she's not young and she's not quiet."

"I'm sorry," she said. "I'll work on it." From there on out, Annie left me alone. It was a good thing for her she agreed to watch herself. I don't know what I would have done if she hadn't.

The next few weeks were a struggle. I was not having a good time and the hours were tough. I wasn't there to front for the cameras. I wasn't there to get more fame. I was really there to win money for sickle cell patients. On the fifth week, I was elected team leader for our group. The challenge involved Loews Hotels, and we were asked to work as hoteliers at Loews Regency in New York. It was actual hard work. We were really doing it. The producers wouldn't let people help you with anything. We had a task where you had to carry a red carpet, so I had to put it on my back and really carry it. It was crazy.

During the Loews challenge, it was my responsibility as project manager to delegate and place all the employees in their roles. Basically, I had to do whatever it took to run a major hotel. And our team won. That meant that I earned $20,000 for the Sickle Cell Foundation of Georgia, which felt really good. But my win was overshadowed by Dennis Rodman, who was the team captain of the opposing group. He'd been behaving erratically and was accused of drinking on the job. Everyone in the boardroom said they thought he was an alcoholic. He got fired that week. So no one said to me, "Congratulations on your win!" It was more like, "Oh, poor Dennis." And yeah, poor Dennis. That sucks. But this wasn't the first time anyone had seen him drunk or seen him not doing what he was supposed to do. But at the end of the day, I won money to help sick children with sickle cell and that's a big accomplishment.

But after that I'd had enough. I was tired, especially since they overworked us and never let us get any sleep. I wanted to go. I'd always chill with the makeup and hair people and with the cameramen, and they'd give me all the dirt on how the show worked. They told me that people could get fired for volunteering to go back into the boardroom because Trump didn't like it. On the sixth week, Donald tasked us with creating viral videos for All laundry detergent. He'd reshuffled the teams, and I'd ended up on one with Jesse James, Annie, Melissa, and Brande. The people from All ended up rejecting both the videos, so no one won. We'd worked 16 hours, and we were scheduled to shoot a double amount of scenes the next day. Nope. That was enough.

The next day was October 20, Chase's birthday. So I was like, "Bump this show. I don't want to be on here anymore. I won't miss these chicks cackling and talking over each other. I did what I came to do, and I'm not going to miss my daughter's birthday for nothing or no one." When Donald called people into the boardroom, Melissa asked us in, which was perfect. How could I not volunteer to join her? Donald was not pleased. Melissa, to her credit, tried to defend me, but Donald said she would have been the one fired if I hadn't volunteered. "Never volunteer for an execution," he told me.

He ended up firing me and Khloé on the same night. He didn't respect her because she had a DUI. It was totally unrelated to the week's task. Typical. But then, Donald was disrespectful. He'd yell at the camera guys, saying things to them like, "Hurry the fuck up!" Right there in front of everyone. It was ugly. I wasn't impressed. It seemed like he had these token people he's cool with and that's it. I got a lot of compliments when I won my challenge, and he seemed so surprised by that. But his opinions didn't pay my bills. I wasn't about to switch up who I was for Donald Trump and some cameras. He couldn't even say my name correctly. He kept messing it up, so after the first week, I told the producers he needed to say it right or abbreviate my name or I was gonna say something about it on national television. He started called me "T," so I assume they passed along the message.

I didn't care about winning by that point. But I wish I could have a do-over when I wasn't sick.

I had to stay in New York for another week to shoot my goodbye scenes. They put you in a car with some cameras and you have to reflect on how it felt to do the show. But on the day after I got fired it was Chase's birthday, and that was the only thing that mattered to me. I took her on a shopping spree to FAO Schwarz and then to Dylan's Candy Bar, and to eat at the Jekyll & Hyde Club. To this day, she says it's one of her favorite birthdays. FAO Schwarz had this place where you could make a Barbie that looks just like you. You could dress it just like you, and your personalized Barbie could do a runway show in the display case afterward. I got one for Chase and she loved it. It was a really cool bonding moment between us.

The real drama happened behind the scenes of that season of *The Celebrity Apprentice*, though. I'd stayed in the Trump International Hotel a bunch of times. Throughout all our tours, TLC had dropped $1 million at that hotel. Seriously, $1 million. But this time, as I was suffering through the show, the maids decided it would be cool to heist a bunch of my jewelry. It was so shady. They really stole my jewelry with my mama and daughter in the room. How bold!

First of all, it doesn't take three or four women to clean a hotel room. But they kept arriving in groups. One of my necklaces, a vintage one-of-a-kind cross, went missing. Another necklace, which I left sitting on the kitchen table, nearly vanished when one of the maids tried to slide it into her pocket as my mama was sitting right there. She missed her pocket and it fell on the floor.

We called the cops right away. When they interviewed the maids, there was a lot of not talking. They pretended not to understand English. The cops said, "Maybe your daughter was playing with the jewelry and misplaced it." No way. Chase knew how to handle diamonds. She knew better than to mess with jewelry because she'd been around nice things since birth. Good try.

I said, "Well, if you ask the maids whether they took my jewelry, they're obviously going to say no." That's like asking a serial killer if he murdered somebody and buried them in Central Park. You think he's just going to say yes? Nothing. No one talked.

Finally, I took matters into my own hands. "Look," I said to the maids. "I know one of you hos understands English. Let me tell you like this: If my jewelry comes back, I will let this go. But if it does not, me and my security will get to y'all. We will come up in your house and take everything I want and I'll beat your ass, too."

Miraculously, by the next day, all my jewelry was returned. Someone had placed it in my mother's walker. Isn't that something?

It was a strange time, but the whole *Celebrity Apprentice*

debacle reminded me that I should take my time getting back to work. I needed to listen better to my body. I was ready to move forward, and I needed to do so in the best way possible.

But sometimes death has a way of worming its way into your life. It's always there as a possibility, but sometimes it arrives without warning. Or, at least, it arrives when you don't expect it to. I'd survived somehow. I'd lived, despite all odds. But not everyone is so lucky.

My cousin Donnie and I grew up together. He was a few years older than me, and he was always my favorite. We'd spend all of our time together when we were younger and whenever we could as adults. When my mama was at work, my aunt Ressie would watch me, and we'd do the silliest things, like standing in the middle of the room, yelling to see who could scream the loudest. My aunt Ressie, who passed away on February 3, 2017, as I was writing this book, was that cool aunt everybody wishes they had. The one who curses and has the funniest conversations. You could eat chocolate cake for breakfast at Auntie Ressie's house. Ressie was everything to me. I loved spending time there with her and Donnie as I was growing up.

Donnie had sickle cell, too. His was sickle cell anemia. He showed a lot of the symptoms and aspects of the disease that I didn't. He had jaundice, yellow eyes, a bloated stomach. He was in a lot of pain a lot of the time. He was always in the hospital. I knew what he was going through, but we were experiencing it differently over the years.

Because Donnie struggled with his disease so much, it meant a lot to me to see him finally have relationships and eventually kids. Even having sex can put you in a crisis because it's like exercise and it strains your body. It can put you in the hospital. It's happened to me. So watching him be able to do some of the normal things that he wasn't always able to do was amazing. Once I convinced him to come visit me in Atlanta and we hung out and went dancing. I just smiled watching him dance because this was a person who had to take a Greyhound from Des Moines to Atlanta because he physically couldn't fly on a plane.

One time Donnie said, "Your pain is worse than mine."

"No," I disagreed. "No way." But it was impossible to know. We both suffered. Sometimes our pain would be so bad we would become delirious and see things. Sometimes the medicine didn't help.

The thing that broke my heart was that Donnie would talk sick and think sick. He bought into the disease and believed it was more powerful than he was.

"Donnie, do you want to come to Atlanta?" I would often ask him on the phone.

"No, I can't right now because I'm gonna be sick," he always replied, even if he wasn't sick at the time. And I feel like if you say you're gonna be sick, then you will be.

In 2009, Donnie had a stroke and got really depressed. He was afraid to move forward or to try new things to treat his disease. Finally I got him to agree to come to Atlanta and try some holistic stuff with Phil, who'd helped me. But right after that Donnie had another stroke and couldn't come. He didn't sound like the cousin I knew anymore. His words slurred. He just wasn't the same.

Donnie's spirit was always happy and bright as we were growing up. He loved music and he loved dancing. He always smiled. But now he sounded so defeated. He fell more and more ill, and he ended up in the hospital. His organs started to fail. It was so bad that the infection spread everywhere in his body, even his genitals. If he stopped breathing and they tried to resuscitate him, he was so weak that his ribs would have broken in half and shattered. So you couldn't even push on his chest.

My mom, who sat by his bedside along with my aunt Ressie, had a pastor come in, just in case. My cousin could rededicate his life to God, just in case.

One day my phone rang. "Tionne," my mama said, "you should get here." But it was the week Chase was supposed to take the standardized tests they force all the kids to take in school. She couldn't miss them. I had to leave her in Atlanta with someone while I flew back to Des Moines to see Donnie, but I couldn't find anyone to watch her and the flights that day were totally booked up. I got in the bathtub with my cell phone and began calling everyone I could think of. I desperately wanted to get there. As I was stepping out of the tub and wrapping myself in a towel, my housekeeper knocked on the door. My landline phone was in her hand.

"Your mother's looking for you," she said. Apparently she hadn't been able to get through on my cell.

"Hello," I said.

"Tionne," she said quietly, "he didn't make it." I froze, still wrapped in a towel.

"Wait a minute," I replied. "What?" I couldn't process it. And I didn't have time to process it. It was Valentine's Day, which I had forgotten about in my scramble to book a flight and find Chase a babysitter. I was supposed to go to this dinner with Takeo and two other couples. It had already been planned, and since I was still in town, I felt like I had to go. I hoped it would help take my mind off the tragedy. I sat at the table and felt like I was there but not there. That night, I stayed at Takeo's. I couldn't sleep. I got out of bed and sat in the bathroom and cried all night. It hit me there in the darkness that Donnie hadn't made it.

My mama told me the story of Donnie's death later, after I had calmed down. You never believe these kinds of stories until you hear them for yourself from someone you really know and trust. She told me that she was lying in Donnie's bed and fell asleep. Aunt Ressie was in the other room, resting. In the middle of the night, my mom felt something touch her arm. When she looked up, it was Donnie. He was smiling at her like he always did. He nodded his head yes, gave her a thumbs-up, and said, "Thank you." And then he disappeared.

As he vanished, Aunt Ressie ran into the room. "I just saw Donnie walk up the hallway," she exclaimed. You can't tell me that two people at the same time didn't see the same person in the same place. My mama told me she believed that Donnie was thanking her for her faith in getting him saved and letting her know that he was okay. And I hope he was.

I didn't get to Des Moines until the funeral. It was awful. Since Donnie and I have the same disease, his death started to mess with my head. I think I wasn't supposed to see him die like that. That would have been so much worse. Everything was preventing me from getting there on time, and now I'm really grateful for that.

I started obsessing. "Am I going to die like that?" I kept

thinking. “Will my death be that way or that bad?” I couldn’t sleep. My nerves were totally shot. My doctor had to give me Valium so I could rest. I kept thinking, “Oh Lord, I’m going to die, too.” I had all these terrible thoughts, all the time after Donnie left us. When I’d watched my grandma die of cancer, it had struck me how dying of cancer is such a horrible way to go. Your insides get all eaten up. But watching Donnie made me realize that my own disease could be that bad, too. I had the same blood as him. I knew sickle cell was ugly, and I knew it could cause an ugly death, but not this ugly. His whole body and all his organs shut down, and there was nothing to do but wait for him to die. That could happen to me, too. It made me sick to my stomach just thinking about it. I wanted to tear my veins out of my body and throw them away.

I have sickle cell and I deal with it every day, but now I wanted to figure out my disease even more than I had in the past. What else could I be doing? How could I help my body so I wouldn’t die like this? It gave me some extra fight. If I couldn’t find a cure, I could at least prolong my life. I did more research and started paying more attention to my body.

So how do you go through life knowing you might die? The common thread in all our journeys is that each one will eventually end. This all stops, period. But here’s the thing: You have to keep living while you can. That’s the bottom line. And in order to do that, you have to find out what your personal strength is.

My personal strength is my daughter—and now my son. For me, that’s the reason I decided, again and again, to get my life together and stay here. I have someone to be here for. I have been determined not to die. I just kept telling myself, “I will not die. I will not die." I busted my ass to be where I am today and to be able to do the things I do today. I have to be able to physically take care of my children. You can decide what it is for yourself that keeps you going. There's always something. There's always a motive to get up and try. You'll always have a reason to stay here.

CHAPTER 12

Bouncing Back

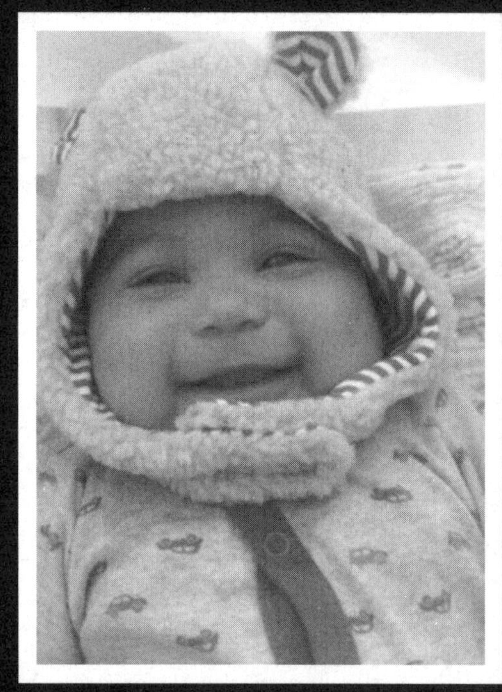

So, now I'd survived a brain tumor, the death of a close friend, the death of a cousin, the death of my grandmother, the death of an aunt, a bad divorce, and life with sickle cell disease. What now? Well, just like with anything, I had to keep living. And if you're born to entertain like me, you have to keep performing.

In 2012, Chilli convinced me that we should tell the story of TLC in a VH1 biopic. We'd been wanting to make something for years when it was still the three of us, but it was never the right time. Now, it was. We worked with a screenwriter named Kate Lanier, and we wanted to give an honest depiction of our journey so far. The good and the bad. Not everything is in there—it's a movie, so some things were generalized—but we were honest about our story.

In the film, directed by Charles Stone III, Lil Mama was cast as Lisa, Keke Palmer as Chilli, and Drew Sidora as me. Chilli and I acted as executive producers, and I worked on some of the choreography, as well. Chase appeared as the younger version of myself in a scene, which worked out since she looks just like me and knows Mommy best. It was strange reflecting back on the band as we made it, but it also reminded me of all our successes. People who had grown up with us could learn the backstory of some of their favorite songs. I recognized the power of that. Plus, people are straight-up nosy. They wanted the dirt behind the scenes.

CrazySexyCool: The TLC Story aired on VH1 on October 21, 2013. An amazing 4.5 million people watched, making it the highest-rated television film premiere of the year and the highest-rated original film premiere on VH1 ever. It got a massive response. Suddenly everyone was talking about TLC again. I even met little girls who thought we were a brand-new group. We released a greatest-hits album, *20*, around the same time, our final release for Epic Records. It had a new song, "Meant to Be," written by Ne-Yo, which appeared in the film.

After the movie came out, some people tried to get their 15 minutes of fame, saying in interviews that they were there with us. But it wasn't anyone else's story to tell. It was from our perspective—it didn't matter who else was in the room.

We had some trouble with Lisa's family, too, when the biopic came out. But let me lay any contention to rest: Only Lisa and I knew our relationship and what it was made of. Sure, there were times when we weren't close or when we fought or when we talked crap about each other, but it was always special between us. No one has the right to say they know our true relationship, except for me. Even during the hard times, Lisa and I had a real bond.

We agreed to perform at the American Music Awards in

November with Lil Mama filling in for Lisa onstage. It was the first time TLC had performed with a guest appearance, and it felt really strange, but the record label and the film producers wanted to see us all together after the film came out. We performed "Waterfalls," which had come out 18 years before. It was sort of a reunion and sort of an homage, and it got us fired up about TLC's music again.

Some fans got confused, thinking we were inducting Lil Mama into the group as a replacement for Lisa. That was never the plan. TLC will always be Chilli, Lisa, and me. There's no changing that. We're not emotionally ready for a hologram, and we will never be ready for a new member. Lil Mama did a great job with Lisa's raps, and we were grateful for the chance to include her in the biopic, but as TLC went forward, we remained the same.

TLC had always wanted to make another album after *3D*. That experience had been tough, and my depression after Lisa died had taken away some of my passion for songwriting. Now, seeing how much the fans still cared, Chilli really wanted to create more music. I was the holdup, but I eventually came around. We'd finally gotten ourselves off Epic Records and Sony at the end of 2013, after the AMAs. There were rumors flying around we'd been dropped from the label, but in reality our contract was just over. After LaFace had folded, TLC had been moved over to Jive Records, which was part of Sony, as well, and then over to Epic with L. A. Reid. We left Sony in late 2013 and ended our merchandising deal with them in 2015. In that deal, we let Forever 21 and H&M sell TLC shirts, which was great because they did amazingly well. Being released from a contract after that long was a real relief. And, more important, we rerecorded all of our old hits from the earlier albums, so now we own the masters. We can license our own version of the songs, so the payday comes to us instead of Sony. Now we had the freedom to do whatever we wanted as artists. We decided to make one final TLC album, our way.

You don't necessarily need a record label anymore. In the past, when we were coming up, record labels were the only way you could get the cash to pay for tours and recording time and other album costs. But in recent years crowdfunding Web sites like Kickstarter have allowed artists to connect directly with fans and make albums for the people. Our manager, Bill, brought it to our attention. Plus, all labels seem good for these days is getting radio play. We had all these fans who were crying out for new music, so Chilli and I figured it was worth trying out Kickstarter to fund our album.

In January of 2015, we launched a Kickstarter page with a long announcement. "We are recording our last and final album," we wrote. "And we want to do it with you, our fans (our babies!). This album, our final album, is dedicated to all of you that have stuck with us, always challenging us to do our best. And of course, it's for the new fans too! We just want to put out great music that touches everyone. That's it." We added, "While major labels offer artists multimillion dollar recording and marketing budgets, they don't often give artists complete control of their own music. It is essential that we create our final album completely on our own terms, without any restrictions, with you." We meant that, too. We wanted to make an album that represented us and no one else. We wanted to do it in our own way.

I was leery of using Kickstarter in the beginning. But

sometimes you have to take chances and we're known for always doing things outside the box. TLC was one of the first artists to do an MP3 deal, and we got a lot of negative comments for it, but when it was successful, people started saying how brilliant it was. When something is new or people don't entirely understand the business of something, they can be afraid to try it—especially in the music industry. No one wants to do anything until it's a proven success. Some thought we were nuts for doing this on Kickstarter.

Our initial goal was $150,000, which would cover an executive producer, other producers, engineers, mixing, mastering, and marketing for the album. We offered a ton of different rewards for the fans who contributed. We wanted to make sure they really felt our gratitude. We've always been a band who has succeeded because of our fans, and this time that feeling was even more significant. In the end, 4,201 backers on Kickstarter pledged $430,255 to bring our album to life—nearly three times our original goal. We broke a record on Kickstarter for the amount raised in the first 2 days. We got support from a ton of fans, including Katy Perry, who pledged $5,000 to get a sleepover with me.

We spent a long time working on the album. Ron Fair acted as our executive producer. It's incredibly hard to book writers and producers. It's also hard to find a new sound. There was a lot of pressure since we're known for making timeless music. I wanted to see if I could deliver it again and if the fans who'd followed us would still love the songs. Plus, we also wanted to make sure we found new fans along the way.

We had a hard time scheduling the writers and producers we wanted to work with. It felt like pulling teeth. It held up the recording process and became really stressful for me and Chilli. My brother Kayo and I own a studio, and we have a lot of writers and producers in and out of there all the time. He had the idea to do a writers camp in Los Angeles, which means you rent out multiple studio rooms for several days to write and then you go room to room to pen songs. It worked. I went every day and worked hard on the new music. My brother ended up being really influential in helping put together the album. He introduced us to some awesome talent. You might think I'd work with my brother only because he's family, but he's legitimately a great producer. And, anyway, I don't believe in homeboy hookups if it's going to jeopardize my career in any way.

A lot of songs came out of the camp. It was such a success. Then Chilli put together a second camp for 2 days in Atlanta, which gave us a few more songs. There was a deadline approaching and the fans were antsy, but we felt we should postpone the initial release because we wanted the music to be right. You can't rush art. Fans don't always realize that there are real reasons for those kinds of delays. I spent hours with Ron perfecting the album and putting my heart into the music. In a lot of ways, it felt like a rebirth of my creativity after several years of heartache and hardship. My brother, who knows me better than anyone, helped produce a lot of the songs on this album, as well.

We'd promised to deliver the record in October of 2015, but in all honesty we needed more time. I also felt like a date shouldn't have been given at that point. We wanted to make sure it felt like a TLC album and that we were true to ourselves as musicians. We ended up with 15 tracks.

People have asked us which of our past albums we'd

compare the new music to, and I don't know how to answer that exactly. I just say it's a TLC album with a TLC sound. That means the songs are relatable and have a catchy tune, with dance routines to support them. Some music doesn't have an age. A good song is a good song and it exists on its own. It can be timeless and classic, and you can remember it forever. Every generation will love it if they like that sort of music. We didn't make new music because we're trying to take advantage of a sense of nostalgia or because we want to remake popular old songs. I'd never try to do something I've already done. I wanted to stay close to the system we've used over the years, but bring in new ideas and new subjects to talk about. We've always been a band who makes universal music that can reach any listener. We don't limit that, and I've never agreed when people have tried to lump us in as rap or R&B. Our music crosses generations and genres, and it's for everyone.

Of course, we came up in the '90s and the '90s were the bomb, so that era will always be part of who we are. The music then was amazing. The music industry was thriving and there was so much talent everywhere. Mega superstars existed. We were able to be part of that. But even as the '90s have faded away, we're still here. I'm still here. TLC has this massive catalogue of timeless music. Our songs are connected to the '90s, but they reach far beyond.

The music industry is hard. I won't try to front and tell you that it's not. It always has been, but it's way worse now. Albums just don't sell like they used to. You have to figure out how to have longevity in this business, which we've done. And even when you do well and you're successful, you still have to learn how to constantly reinvent yourself. You have to always be aware of why fans liked you in the first place. What did you do right and how can you evolve from there? What could you do differently next time that will help push you forward? How does one stay relevant in a dishonest industry? And how can you survive financially without being taken advantage of?

The truth is that the music business is never going to be the same again. Streaming has changed how we listen to music. Record labels are dying. Social media is essential. There are more artists making more music, and listeners are really discerning. But ultimately, fans still want good music. They still want to go to concerts and sing along to music that means something to them.

Here's what I know now about being a performer: You can't underestimate yourself or sell yourself short. There are people in this industry who will want to control you and who will try to force you to use your sexuality in a way that male performers never have to. There will be female artists who take their clothes off and think that's the best way to sell records. I don't have a problem with that, but it's not my way of doing things as an artist. And you don't have to do that. TLC had success by being ourselves and never compromising who we were. Being a woman in music is a strike against you, and being a black woman, another strike. If you buy into the idea that girls need to get butt-naked onstage or on TV to make it or be successful, well, it's just not true. I've worked for what I've achieved, and I haven't taken my pants off to do it.

If you want to be a musician—or an artist of any kind—it's important to learn about the business you're in. Because it is a business. You're here to make art *and* to make money, and unfortunately those things go hand in hand most of the time. It's not even really the music business anymore—it's the entertainment business. It's become so much more now that reality TV has taken over. Do your research and learn how it all works. Read your contracts before you sign them, and really make sure you understand what's on those pages. Some lawyers and accountants can have their own agenda. How will it affect you 10 years—or even 20 years—down the line? Work with people you trust and who respect you. Respect yourself, too. Don't let anyone tell you that you can't do something if you know you can.

My mom always told me I could be anything I wanted to be as long as I had good morals, integrity, and character, and if I worked hard. She never doubted me when I said I was meant for the spotlight, and I've never doubted any of Chase's dreams either. You need people in your life who support you and who believe in you. And, most important, you have to believe in yourself. My mom held my hand when I got sick, and she held it when I triumphed in TLC. I want to do the same for my children. I can tell you for sure that it's possible to overcome any odds. You might think you can't get to the top because of where you're from or what your background is, but that's just not true. Three black girls living in Atlanta became the highest-selling girl group of all time, which should tell you that color and gender and class don't matter. What matters is who you are inside.

If you stand behind your work and speak your mind, it will always mean something to your fans. I've learned to be careful how I say things and to be mindful of the best way to express myself, too. It matters how you say something as much as it does what you say. It's been amazing for me to see how many people have been touched by TLC's music over the years. When I wrote "Unpretty," I wasn't thinking that it would be a massive song; I was trying to express what I was feeling at the time. It turned out that a lot of people felt that same thing or had shared my sentiments at some point in their life. My song gave them a way to relate. It made them feel less alone, which is the most important thing music can do. To me, personal songs are the ones that work best.

When we were working on our greatest-hits album in 2013, Dallas asked me to come into the studio to meet Lady Gaga because she'd written a song for TLC called "Posh Life." I didn't know she was a fan, but when I got to the studio, she grabbed my hand and said, "Oh my God, I can't believe it." She was so passionate about the music we'd made. She told me that she'd really connected to "Unpretty" when she was growing up.

"You don't understand how much that song helped me," she told me, in tears. "You helped me so much. I was an outcast, but you made me feel like I was good enough to fit in because of what you sang and wrote. You made me feel good about myself."

"But you're Lady Gaga," I said, surprised. "My daughter loves you."

"I know and I appreciate that," she replied. "But I'm a fan. You've changed my life."

She was like a kid, so excited to be meeting me. She cried because TLC was so important to her. That meant the world to me. And we've had so many fans express similar emotions. We've had people tell us that our music saved their life. You never know who you're going to reach, which is why I love music so much. "Posh Life" never ended up being on the album because of some political issues, but it gave me the chance to meet a fellow artist whose life had changed because of something I wrote. How lucky. Although it never came out, recording "Posh Life" and knowing that Lady Gaga wrote it was satisfaction enough.

Over the past 2 years, TLC has kept touring. We toured the US with New Kids on the Block and Nelly, and we trekked to Japan, New Zealand, and Australia to headline arenas. We played music festivals around the country and met old and new fans alike. People still scream our name when we come onstage and as we leave, except this time they're all waving cell phones in the air, trying to capture Snapchats and Instagram posts of "Waterfalls." I get to see how much we still mean to fans every month, which keeps me going.

I don't know what the future of TLC will be beyond our new album. I like the idea of doing a residency show somewhere like Las Vegas. I've written some solo material. I think our songs will endure, even when TLC no longer makes any new music. We've broken records, and our band has given me everything I have today. I don't take that lightly. I will always be the T in TLC, no matter what.

As the world of TLC has changed, so has my life at home. Having Chase was one of the most miraculous things that's happened to me. If you ask me my greatest achievement, I'll still say Chase. She was so unexpected and amazing. She made me a new person, took away some of my anger, and gave me a reason to keep pushing through any sickle cell crisis or tragedy. But because I have this disease, I've always wondered if I'd be able to give her a sibling. It's unclear, especially at my age, whether I can have another child. For years, I've wanted a son. Luckily, there's more than one way to make a family.

I'd thought about adopting for years. I was devastated by the news of the 2010 earthquake in Haiti, and for a while, I wondered if I could adopt a child in need from there. An opportunity for me to adopt a 2-year-old baby from Iowa came up. I was so excited. I bought toys and clothes and started preparations for him to join my life. But it wasn't meant to be. When it came time to go to the lawyer's office to sign the papers, the birth mother didn't show. I was devastated. But I also think that everything happens for a reason.

TLC was scheduled to do a few days of press in New York ahead of our tour with New Kids on the Block. We woke up super early to tape *Good Morning America*, much earlier than my body wanted to be awake. After the show aired, my mama called. "Tionne," she said, "you looked puffy." She didn't mean fat. She meant I looked swollen and sick. I looked in the mirror. She was right. My face was puffing up. When I got home to LA, I started feeling a sharp pain under my left breast. It hurt every time I lay down, every time I got up, and every time I took a breath. But I kept on with my day. I have a high tolerance for pain so sometimes I don't realize how sick I really am. My brother said, "Go to the ER." But I didn't want to. I hate being poked with needles because I have so few working veins. They can use the ones in my feet and the ones in my neck, but usually those have to be reserved for emergencies. Lately, the only veins that seem to work are the ones in my breast.

Instead of going to the ER, I went to tape my radio show. The pain got worse. It spread down my entire side. Every breath I took hurt. I couldn't take it anymore. I called Chase and she packed a bag and we headed to the hospital. It took them three tries to get an IV in my arm.

"Ms. Watkins," someone said, "we're going to roll you in an ER room and check you out for a few things." I waited in there for a while and then a doctor showed up.

"Ms. Watkins, we're waiting for this room to become available in the ICU," he told me. "We're going to take you up there now." The ICU? I knew what it had to be. This pain was familiar.

"Is it my spleen?" I asked him.

"I'm not allowed to tell you that," he replied.

"You're not telling me," I said. "I'm telling you and I'm asking if it's my spleen." He nodded. I knew it. And I was furious. A tear rolled down my cheek, but I couldn't fully cry because Chase was there and I didn't want to upset her. I was angry because I'd been doing so well. I'd been eating right. I'd been trying all these new holistic remedies. I'd been on track. But then we had to go to New York and the schedule was so hectic and rigorous that it messed up my health. I should never have to get up that early for morning shows and work all day and night. My body needs time to adjust to the different time zones, and I need my team to plan a better schedule with my health in mind, because my body can't handle it. I'd told everyone the schedule was too much, which it clearly was, and now I was sick again. I'd let people put me in situations I shouldn't be in. It really pissed me off.

I started to think about the baby I wasn't able to adopt. Maybe I couldn't keep him because I was going to be sick. Maybe I wasn't supposed to have him because I was going to die. My mind spiraled.

The doctors, who were not my usual doctors, started

talking about removing my spleen completely. Dr. Braunstein called from Atlanta. "Do not take out her spleen," he instructed. "Her spleen may be dead tissue, but she has accessory spleens."

That meant that I had small extra spleens growing on the outside of my dead one. Think about that. It's pretty incredible. My body was compensating. I could still fight off viruses and colds if I had these accessory spleens. The doctors followed Dr. Braunstein's orders and I was able to heal without surgery. Now I have to fight to keep these baby spleens. If you think my immune system is bad now, imagine what it would be like without them.

A few months later, while TLC was on tour with New Kids on the Block, I had a realization. I was sitting on the tour bus talking to my hairstylist Chris.

"I have to figure out if I am going to adopt or have a surrogate or get a sperm donor," I said. "But I need do to something. I'm 45 and I want a boy."

After all I've been through, I don't ever want to feel like I woulda, coulda, shoulda about anything. I could get to 60 and regret never having a second kid in my life and that would suck. You can't ever get a do-over. So I decided, "Let's do this. Life is short and I'm going to make the most of it." There's never a perfect time to expand your family, especially when you're a traveling performer. When I had Chase, I said, "I'll figure this out." And now I would figure out how to work my life around a teenager and an infant at the same time. You make do and you try your best. Any parent will tell you that.

A few days later I was with my mama. She called me over to her and told me to sit down.

"I want to talk to you about something," she said. I nodded.

"Remember the baby you were going to adopt?" she said. "His mother is pregnant again and wants you to have this baby." Was she serious? I'd gotten so emotionally attached and bought all this stuff the first time around. I didn't want to go through that again. "She's serious," my mama continued, reassuring me. "This is it."

So I decided to try again. Adoption is an incredibly difficult process. It's stressful and emotionally draining and it wears on every last nerve. There's social workers and so much paperwork. It's really invasive. They ask you so many questions. It's exhausting. I had to take a 6-hour class to become certified in CPR and first aid. I also took online courses that I had to pass. People write letters about you and seal them up, so you can't ever see what's written. Social workers come to your house and check everything. They go through your personal belongings. They test your smoke detectors. Everyone in the house, including the dog, has to get TB shots. The adoption agency compiles everything into a massive file. There is so much involved, and it all feels very precarious. Chance was appointed a lawyer that they called a guardian who was yet another person who came and watched my interaction with my son. I didn't mind that but it was just that the opinions of these people determined whether I got to keep him or not once I went to court.

It's just so scary. You get attached and you actually have the baby and the thought that the court could still take the baby back was terrifying. It would have broken my heart. And it's very expensive. But it's worth it.

I wasn't allowed to be there for the baby's birth. My mom went as the custodian. Chase and I watched over FaceTime. Chase is a happy crier, so she was bawling the whole time. I was excited, but I didn't want to let myself feel too much. I was allowed to name him and make all his medical decisions with the doctors, but he wasn't quite mine yet. And what if it didn't work out? There's a waiting period where the birth mother can still change her mind. My son was here in the world, and I couldn't touch him. My mom sent photo after photo. I was happy, but my heart hurt at the same time. But finally, 9 days after his birth, I was allowed to meet my new son.

He was so tiny and so beautiful. To me, he was perfect. He looked just like Chase. It seemed impossible that he could look that much like her. He took to me instantly. My mom and my aunt Ressie had been with him for the past 9 days, and they watched him with me. They noticed that he stopped crying when I held him. "He knows you're his mommy," my mama said. My pediatrician once told me that babies can feel love. I wasn't sure if he could feel what was coming from my heart, but my love for him was so strong. He leaned against my heart, just like Chase had when she was born, and suddenly I knew he felt it, too.

I was going to name him Cayo because I'd been watching *Naked and Afraid* on the Discovery Channel and it was set in Cayo, Mexico. But no one else liked it. "Everyone is going to think his name is Kyle," my mom informed me. "And everyone is going to make fun of him at school because it sounds like the cartoon *Caillou*," my niece added. But Chase had an idea. "How about Chance?" she said. "You were going to name me that, and it goes perfectly with Chase." So I named him Chance Ace Watkins.

I had to stay with Chance in Iowa until a judge held a court date for his biological parents. They had to completely give up their parental rights. It was nerve-racking to wait for that day to come. I worried that they'd change their mind and take him away from me. I was cleared to take him home with me, but then the judge moved the court date back, giving them more time to change their mind, which stressed me out. I couldn't stay in Iowa much longer because Chase was in school back in California. The court date finally arrived. The papers were signed and no one changed their mind. Another hurdle crossed. Carrying Chance into our home was a huge moment. He got to come home, to the place I hoped he'd be for years to come.

Next we had to wait for my own court date. Chance and I returned to Iowa in May of 2016, 9 months after he was born.

"Why do you think he should remain yours?" the judge asked me.

"Your Honor," I said, "I have this box of boy's baby clothes. I've been keeping it for years. I always said my son would wear those clothes and that's my son. I spoke him into existence and that's him." I burst into tears. I meant it so fiercely. The judge awarded him to me officially, and it was strange because I felt the same way then that I did when Chase was born. It was a feeling of pure and absolute joy.

Chance is a true blessing to me and to our family. He's brought new life and fulfillment in our house and made us feel even more complete, and I can't thank his biological parents enough for bringing him into this world. He gives me yet another thing to live for.

Lately, my health continues to fluctuate. Sometimes I'm healthy and sometimes my disease rears its ugly head. With all I do to remain healthy, I don't get sick as much as I used to. My trips to the hospital have lessened. My organs push through. I still have some side effects that linger from the brain surgery. My smile may always be slightly crooked. I still struggle with pain. But I've survived so much. I have outlived several death sentences, and thank God for that. I eat better and avoid situations of stress or high altitude or cold. I take holistic remedies daily and try new ones to see if they work. I take myself to that place of peace and calm, where three waterfalls join a river. I take myself on a boat down the stream to a beautiful big ocean. I quiet myself and try to remember, "This pain won't last forever."

Life is tough. And for many years I've felt like I've worked to get sick and worked to get better, just to get sick again. I'm learning to find a balance and just live. You lose people and you fall ill and bad things can happen. But it's also really miraculous. You can have babies you were told you'd never have. You can bring joy to millions of people with your music. You can feel love and happiness and faith. You can decide that you're stronger than any obstacle and you can empower yourself to survive. I know things can get really dark, but you'll always feel better if you hold on. The light always returns. You can't let anyone tell you otherwise. It's like my mama told me when I was 7: God has the final say-so in your life. You have to keep pushing forward, smiling, and walking with your head up.

My life, my sick life, has been tinged with illness. But I refuse to be defined by it. I don't need to walk around every day like a patient. I've got too much to do. I've always kept standing up, again and again, no matter what obstacle was placed in front of me, and I will keep doing that for as long as it is humanly possible. I have so much to live for and so do you. I don't know what's coming next, but I do know that I can handle it. They say that God doesn't put more on your plate than you can take on, and I agree.

Ultimately, you have to find something positive to believe in, whatever it is. For me, it's God. For you, it might be something else. Take whatever is stressing you out or making you feel negative, and get rid of it. The mind can be a powerful tool and so can words. I think you can speak things into existence. Voice what you want. You have the capacity to ask for it.

Like I told the judge, I used to keep that box of boy baby clothes in my house, long before Chance arrived into my life. I knew what I wanted, and I knew it was possible before it ever happened. I have my son, and he has those clothes. Now Chance, Chase, and I, just like TLC, were MTB.

ACKNOWLEDGMENTS

Thank you to my amazing mother who loves me unconditionally and raised me to become the woman I am today!

My children are my life and why I keep going, no matter what!

Thanks to all family and friends for supporting me.

Thanks to Kayo and Brian for believing in me.

Thanks to the fans because it's impossible to do without you.

Thanks to Emily Zemler, Laura Nolan, Mark Sacro, and the people at Rodale. I'd like to express my gratitude to the many people who saw me through this book, providing support, talking things over, reading, writing, and assisting with the editing, proofreading, and design.

And thanks to God who has been with me and saw me through everything! I praise God that I'm so blessed to have the opportunity to share a part of my life.

INDEX

An asterisk (*) indicates photos shown in color inserts.